# THE
# SATISFICERS

# THE
# SATISFICERS

## ARTHUR LEVIN, M. D.

*The McCall Publishing Company*

NEW YORK

*Published simultaneously in Canada by*
*Doubleday Canada Ltd., Toronto.*

*Library of Congress Catalog Card Number: 74–137678*

*SBN 8415-0054-1*

*The McCall Publishing Company*
*230 Park Avenue, New York, N.Y. 10017*

PRINTED IN THE UNITED STATES OF AMERICA

*Design by Tere LoPrete*

Officials do not try to maximize but, instead, they "satisfice" (satisfy and suffice). Which is to say that they do not try for the best of all possible worlds . . . they try to "get by," to "come out all right," to "avoid trouble," to "avoid the worst," and so on.

AARON WILDAVSKY

# CONTENTS

# Introduction by
# Senator George McGovern

Among the most curious anomalies of contemporary American life is the appalling job we do in securing the health of our citizens. In my role as chairman of the Select Committee on Nutrition and Human Needs, I have seen the toll taken by our inability—and too often our unwillingness—to feed the hungry poor of this land. Hunger, as we have become so vividly aware, does not exist in isolation. The hungry poor are also the homeless poor, the jobless poor, the frightened unprotected poor, and, most dramatically, the sick poor. Their children are born earlier and smaller and more of them die in infancy; those who survive are more often sick and seriously disabled; they are stunted in mental and physical development; and their deaths come earlier.

But these are not the only Americans for whom health care is inadequate. Even the very wealthy, who can take advantage of the sophisticated advances in medical science, may not have access to it. For most Americans health care is something obtained only at great cost and enormous inconvenience, and then with little assurance of the most rudimentary protection against unreasonable prices and unsafe medicines.

What was written as an account of one young man's sojourn in the federal health establishment turns out to be a sweeping indictment of the federal agencies most responsible for health care. Dr. Levin has written an entirely personal record of his experience as a noncareer, commissioned officer in the U.S. Public Health Service. He provides an insider's glimpse into the process that denies adequate health care to millions of Americans every day. It will come as small comfort to realize that poor health care is not a matter of specific policy but of bureaucratic incompetence, and inertia. This deadly combination, Dr. Levin tells us, adding a new word to the lexicon of bureaucracy, leads everyone to "satisfice"—an amalgam of satisfy and suffice—and this results in a safe bureaucracy that does as little as possible.

It requires little imagination to understand—after reading this book—why we find ourselves in the midst of a national health crisis. It requires no effort at all to appreciate how such pressing human concerns as hunger and medical care can "fall between the cracks." Dr. Levin does us all a service in sharing his vantage point with those of us whose taxes support, but whose needs are only poorly represented in, the health bureaucracies of our federal government.

# FOREWORD

The events in this book, in which the author—almost by accident—was privileged to participate, took place at a perplexing time in our history. They occurred at a time when, despite general affluence, our social structure seemed to be on the verge of chaos. They occurred when, despite passage of more new social legislation than at any other comparable period in the nation's history, social progress seemed stymied. They happened at a time when, despite an ever-growing awareness of social problems, less and less seemed to be able to be done to solve them.

This is a book about the men and women who run our government's social programs. It is the story of their attempts to plan, operate, and occasionally to judge how well these programs are working. It is the story of how they perceive and respond to events beyond their marble-encased windows—to the complaint of a man in Pennsylvania, to a congressman's tirade, or to the angry demands of the poor.

More important, this is also the story of the things these men and women who run our social programs don't do—the decisions and actions they do not make or take. It is the story of the issues they cannot solve and purposely muddle. It is a chronicle of the developing problems they chose to overlook, of mandates they fail to carry out, and of judgments they fail to exercise. It is the story of individuals, and the organizations they represent, dedicated both through necessity and inclination to one principle: in order to survive—in the inimitable jargon of the bureaucracy—they must only "satisfice."

Much of this book, it should be noted, could not have been written before the recently enacted Truth in Government law. Many episodes have been pieced together from verbatim transcripts of government meetings or from memoranda which, previously, would have been classified "administrative confidential" and thus not for public release. The law now requires that these documents be made available, upon request, to citizens, although many of these documents are still inaccessible for the simple reason that federal officials probably could not locate them even if asked to do so. They have disappeared in the shifting sands of the bureaucracy. Other episodes are reconstructed from notes of my own, since following the enactment of the Truth in Government law many officials put an end to the practices of keeping minutes or transcripts of official meetings.

Government officials, even the worst, are no better nor worse than other people. They are subject to the same motivations and predilections. This book is meant, not as criticism of any particular official, but as a portrayal of an entire institution and the attitudes of certain people within it. Although the government might benefit from the removal of one or more individuals who now hold important positions in it, this would not automatically guarantee any improvement in the manner in which the government reacts to social problems. For this reason, I have occasionally altered the names of persons or, less frequently, withheld certain details by which they might be identified, in order to hinder those who might be interested in vindictive action against any official still working for a federal agency. With this single qualification, all the events described were actual situations in which actual people— including the author—played their respective roles.

In writing this book I have been immeasurably aided by many individuals concerned with the broad panorama of social change and national potential. In particular, I am indebted to George and Mitzi Silver for the many personal kindnesses they showed me during my stay in Washington and for their constant encouragement during the period in which this book was being written. I have also profited from my association with many others in Washington, among whom I would especially like to mention Ruth Covell, Phillip Lee, Joseph Wholey, James and Peggy King, Mancur Olson, Robert Grosse, Sid Johnson, George Deming, and William Anderson. Nancy Amidei deserves special thanks for her helpful criticism of the chapter on hunger and malnutrition.

This book is for these men and women who, by occupation and inclination, spend much of their time thinking about the social tasks our nation has yet to complete. It is for these day-to-day workers who toss the rivets and clamber among the girders of an unfinished America, that this book is written.

# THE
# SATISFICERS

# CHAPTER

## 1

# *While Washington Burned*

Late one afternoon in the spring of 1968, just before the Poor People's Campaign, I attended a meeting in the office of one of HEW's assistant secretaries. The meeting had been arranged to discuss ways of evaluating the department's programs to see how well they were working. The assistant secretary opened it with a short speech. He stressed the urgent need for a concerted effort to find out how well Health, Education, and Welfare's massive social programs were working—an effort that had never been made before.

The department didn't really know, he said, how well its educational programs were helping children to learn or its training programs helping people get jobs. It hadn't ever really tried to find out if its health programs were helping to diminish illness and disability. The task, he said, was to get this sort of information on all of HEW's programs.

Everyone seemed to think that the idea of seeing how well the department's programs were working was a good one. But no one could agree on how it was to be done.

"Let's contract the job out to RAND, or to anyone who will do it," someone suggested.

Someone else objected. The problem was, he said, that RAND—or any of the other "think tanks"—knew nothing about how government social programs operated. "By the time they learn enough about education or health," he said, "we could have done the job ourselves."

Another official argued that HEW simply didn't have enough skilled persons—economists, statisticians, and just plain bright people—to do the job. The time spent teaching the RAND "whiz kids" about education or health, he maintained, would be time and money well spent.

"Who knows," he said. "Maybe we can even convince some of them to come and work here instead of working on a better missile system for the Defense Department."

"Didn't RAND offer us a proposal?" someone asked.

"Yes. For half a million bucks." There was a gloomy silence.

The meeting dragged on. No one could seem to agree on how the evaluation plan should proceed. The hour was late and my attention wandered. I found myself gazing out of the assistant secretary's picture window at the city. From my seat opposite the window I could see almost all of Washington. A thin sliver of the Capitol's dome still gleamed in the setting sun, the remainder in eclipse. Suddenly my eyes focused on something beyond and just to the left of the dome—something that made it look small by comparison.

"Look," said someone else, at almost the same moment my eyes became aware of this extraordinary addition to the skyline. "Look at that."

Everyone's attention turned toward the window. An immense cloud of black smoke was rising behind the Capitol, from the area of Washington's commercial section. In the peaceful stillness of the assistant secretary's luxurious office the rising cloud seemed almost unreal, some theatrical trick or magical apparition. Someone whistled. No one said anything.

The telephone rang and the assistant secretary jumped to answer it.

"Business is over," he said. "The city is burning. Everyone is to evacuate the building immediately."

The wave of civil disorder that had swept the nation had finally reached Washington. We all stood transfixed by this strange spectacle, like men viewing a rare natural disaster from the protection of a great distance. Only this disaster was man-made. This slowly rising black cloud was the work of human hands.

The reaction of the government—at least that small portion of it I observed—was as undramatic as the sight outside was spectacular. Secretaries quietly locked their desks, covered their typewriters, and left. A few sporadic telephone calls came through and then the phones were silent. Officials lingered at the window for a few moments, as though to make certain that the phenomenon was real, then packed their attaché cases and slowly walked toward the elevators in groups of three or four. Perhaps somewhere someone was busily hiding secret documents or securing the building from attack, but I did not see any such precautions. All I saw were people talking in hushed, solemn tones or just quietly going home like disappointed fans whose favorite baseball team has just lost an important game.

I went to my office and haphazardly stuffed a few papers into my briefcase. It seemed meaningless to think of taking home any work, as I usually did. I took the plan for evaluating HEW's social programs that had been distributed at the afternoon meeting. This too struck me as ludicrous. It seemed at though, in a sense, the ultimate evaluation was at that moment being performed. The careful plans of the officials and "analysts"—their academic discussions of program inputs and outputs—all seemed unreal and inconsequential in the shadow of that horrible cloud behind the Capitol.

Washington was being set afire. The city was burning in a year of unparalleled prosperity, of rising profits and a climbing Gross National Product—the final year of an administration that had written more social legislation than any other in the nation's history. Perhaps this was why the government officials seemed so subdued and morose in the face of this macabre spectacle. Their city was in flames and they did not understand why.

I stood for a moment beside my car in the HEW parking lot, watching the city. Sirens sounded everywhere. A jeep full of national guardsmen, their bayonets fixed, careened around the corner and stopped short. Its occupants looked at me for an instant, then raced away again. Two of my co-workers appeared. One was a woman physician, the other a young man whose family lived in nearby Virginia.

"Would you like to have dinner at my parents' place?" the man asked, as though the thought had just occurred to him.

I agreed. Our car joined the caravan crawling across the Fourteenth Street Bridge toward the safety of the suburbs. The rush-hour traffic was much worse than usual that evening.

"A group of young doctors are organizing to treat riot victims tonight," said the woman physician, "and I've promised that you and I would help. Can you come?"

I replied that I would.

We returned to the city later that evening. The usually fresh night air was heavy with the smell of smoke. An armed guardsman stopped us at the Francis Scott Key Bridge. I fumbled with my wallet and handed him my government identification card that certified that I was a member of the secretary's staff. He looked at it carefully. Then he walked over to a jeep and showed the card to another guardsman. Finally he returned, handed me the card, and waved us on. As we drove away from the checkpoint I saw him stop another car.

A private home served as headquarters for the emergency medical effort. From there volunteer doctors and medical supplies were dispatched to jails and police precincts throughout the city. The scene was one of leisurely chaos.

Two telephones rang constantly with requests for assistance of one sort or another. No single person seemed fully aware of the goings on of the entire operation.

"Wait here in the living room," said the young man who greeted us. "We already have more than enough people out. If anyone asks to be relieved, we'll send you."

We sat in the living room. A plate of cold hors d'oeuvres was passed. An hour went by, but our help didn't seem needed. I was eager to drive downtown in order to see first-hand what was happening, but I thought it too soon to suggest leaving. A fellow engaged us in conversation and asked where we worked.

"Hey," he shouted to some others who were finishing the hors d'oeuvres. "These two work for the secretary of HEW."

"Can't you help us?" someone asked. "We could use another station wagon."

"And a small truck," said another.

"And some supplies."

I looked at my colleague.

"We're sorry," she said quietly, "but we don't have the authority to obtain anything like that for you."

"What do you mean?" one man asked. "You work for the secretary of HEW and you can't do anything for us?"

"We don't actually operate any program," my colleague tried to explain. "We just plan for the future."

Our questioners looked skeptical and disappointed. They went back to their hors d'oeuvres. Soon afterward we left as inconspicuously as possible. Outside the smell of smoke was still heavy and tiny pieces of soot fell in black flakes. There was a reddish glow in the sky over downtown Washington. I turned to my companion.

"You know," I said, "they didn't believe what you told them, but it's true. There's absolutely nothing we can do."

"It's not just us," she replied. "There's nothing anyone, even the secretary himself, can do now. All anyone can do is to begin to develop plans for next year."

# CHAPTER
# 2

## *A Lesson in Blurring an Issue*

The burning of Washington occurred after I had been in the Capitol almost two years. I had come to think of myself—in that city of transients—as a Washingtonian. My world was the world of the government. It was the world of conferences, memoranda, congressional hearings, and urgent White House requests. My world was a Washington far removed from the dance halls of Fourteenth Street or the tenements across the Anacostia River, in a part of the city I'd never visited. The burning of Washington made me think back to the odd, almost accidental events that had brought me there, to that city whose major "industry"—the Government —seemed as far distant from the lives of its citizens as the most insular university.

On January 22, 1966, I was appointed a commissioned officer in the United States Public Health Service. At the time, I was working as an intern at the Boston City Hospital, a huge municipal hospital that serves as vendor for most of the health care dispensed to Boston's poor. Many of my fellow interns had already been drafted into one or another branch of the military service. Some had been ordered to duty in Vietnam. Others were being sent to work in Federal prisons or in Indian hospitals in the Southwest. One was sent to serve on an icebreaker in the Arctic. Still others had jobs as researchers in government laboratories or were going to military bases in the United States. To my surprise, my orders read to report for duty as a "special projects officer" to the Washington offices of the Department of Health, Education and Welfare.

Although I could not help but be surprised—and elated—at having received such a desirable assignment, I knew that it had little to do with any special qualifications I possessed. It had been pure luck. A few months before I'd been eating lunch in the hospital cafeteria when an older man took a seat across the table. I hardly recognized him, though he looked vaguely familiar. He was, he told me, an assistant professor at the Harvard Medical School. We struck up a conversation.

"What will you do after your internship?" he asked me.

"I don't know. I've been so busy I hadn't given it much thought."

"What," he asked, "have you done about the draft—about military service?"

"I was hoping it would go away."

"Well it won't," he said, as though he thought I'd seriously considered the possibility. "Are you at all interested in administrative medicine—in thinking about health problems rather than treating sick people?"

I thought for a moment. "I don't know," I replied. The possibility had never really crossed my mind.

"Let's try to find out," he said, wolfing the remains of his sandwich. We left the cafeteria, crossed the courtyard, and took the elevator to his office. He thumbed through a card catalogue of names and addresses, selected one card, and picked up the phone.

"This fellow used to work with me in the epidemic intelligence service during the war," he said as he waited for the connection. "Now he's in Washington."

I heard a voice answer on the other end of the line.

"Hello, Dick. Jim. Listen. I've got a young man here with a very good record who wants to find out if he's interested in working with you for a while." There was a silence as the voice on the other end answered.

"Fine," said my companion. "Monday?" He turned to me. "Monday all right for you?"

I nodded my head affirmatively.

The following Monday I found myself sitting in a spacious Washington office. Facing me was a middle-aged man in a business suit who was, I gathered, one of the senior officials of the Public Health Service.

"Our office," he said, "acts as the staff for the surgeon general. We help prepare the materials he needs to make decisions. Not too many people," he went on, "realize who the surgeon general is, or how important he is. They don't realize that he has the responsibility for the health of the entire nation. It's our job to help him exercise that responsibility."

The entire interview seemed to take place as though in a motion picture. My interviewer, an extraordinarily handsome man, seemed to be reading from a script, as he explained the functions of his office. It was clear that he had spoken the same piece many times before. Finally he began to talk about my own problem.

"You can satisfy your military service—or draft—requirement by accepting a commission in the Public Health Service. That means you will work for the Public Health Service for two years instead of, say, for the Army or some other branch of the military. We have many doctors each year who satisfy the draft in this way. Of course," he cautioned, "there is no guarantee that you will be assigned to this particular office. But," he added, "we'll do our best to get you on board.

"You should," he concluded, "complete your application as soon as possible. Be sure to put my name on it."

I assured him I would. As I left his office the flag of the Public Health Service caught my eye. It showed a huge gold anchor on a blue background, a symbol, my host told me, of the early days of the service when its main function was to provide health care for merchant seamen. I wondered about the strange circumstances that in the space of a few days had brought me to Washington. I felt a great relief that —in all probability—my application would be acted upon favorably and that I would be assigned to this office. Yet, at the same time, I felt that there was an element of favoritism and string-pulling in the entire process that seemed distasteful. I mentioned this feeling to one of my fellow interns when I returned to Boston.

"Why let it bother you," he said. "Everyone knows that the draft is unfair. It's not as though you're doing anything illegal. You've just stumbled onto a way to get a good deal from the system. Consider yourself lucky—and forget it."

I took his advice, half-convinced that something would go wrong and, like most of my friends, I would be assigned to a Coast Guard cutter or to a remote federal military base. I was truly surprised when, a few months later, my official commission arrived.

"The President of the United States," the engraved document said, "reposing special trust and confidence" in my "patriotism, valor, fidelity, and abilities" was appointing me an officer in the Public Health Service. "This officer," the document's script went on, "will therefore carefully and diligently discharge the duties of the office to which appointed by doing and performing all manner of things thereunto belonging." The words must be exactly the same, I wryly imagined, for someone being sent to one of the battle zones of Vietnam. The document was signed by the surgeon general. The lower left-hand corner bore the gold seal of the Department of Health, Education and Welfare, of which the Public Health Service was part.

I arrived in Washington one sweltering July day, six months later, having been given no idea whatsoever of what the duties of my appointed office were to be. The man who had interviewed me several months before, I learned, was no longer there. He had been reassigned to another post, apparently leaving no instructions with his successor as to what, if anything, I had been brought "on board" to do. The office to which I'd been assigned, its new director somewhat grandiosely told me, now aspired to the responsibility for health "policy planning" for the entire Department of Health, Education and Welfare. My job, I was told, would be that of a "policy analyst."

Like most educated people who have never worked in government, I had only the vaguest notion of what policy was, let alone how to analyze it. I knew virtually nothing about how the federal government worked. With some trepidation, I wondered whether I was destined to spend two years behind a desk doing routine administrative tasks.

One of the first people I met in Washington was the young man who occupied the adjoining office, a prefabricated cubicle exactly like mine. Like me, he was supposed to be a policy analyst, specializing in health matters. He was also, I found out, a part-time Episcopalian minister to a parish located on the outskirts of Washington's Negro neighborhood—if a city that is four-fifths black can be said to have a Negro "neighborhood." He invited me to a tea at the church one Sunday afternoon.

"You won't feel out of place," he reassured me. "The folks who belong to my church are all BASPS—Black Anglo-Saxon Protestants. They're more conservative than William Buckley."

The people at the tea were, indeed, very strait-laced. There were many portly women in silk-print dresses and men in dark-brown suits that looked too heavy for the warm Washington weather. One man in particular seemed highly intrigued by his pastor's weekday job as a policy analyst for the Public Health Service.

"Your work must be most inspiring," he said, taking a deep breath. "Health is so important to everyone. Isn't it wonderful," he went on, "how much longer we can expect to live today than when I was a boy? Do you think, Father, that our life span will soon reach the biblical four score and ten years?"

My friend looked at the man somewhat amused, I thought, at his pomposity.

Then he looked at me for an instant and smiled.

"I think," he said, "that we live just as long as we decide to. Our life span is a social policy decision, just like our unemployment rate or the date of our moon landing. There's really no difference at all. Our nation can have as long a life expectancy as its citizens choose."

His listener looked at him, first with sheer disbelief and then in utter confusion. He mumbled something about the discoveries of science multiplying daily and melted back into the crowd. Later, when the tea was over, I asked my friend if he really believed in his singularly unspiritual view of social progress.

"Maybe there's something of the oversell in what I said," he replied, "but there's more truth in it than you'd imagine. The speed of social progress is determined by our ability to decide what we want. Come to our meeting next week on the kidney machine. You'll see what I mean."

The following week I attended the meeting he had mentioned. The participants were government officials and advisers. The purpose of the meeting was for HEW officials to get advice on timely health problems. All the participants were men and women with years of experience in running public or private programs that sought to "help people" in one way or another. All, I am certain, considered themselves thoughtful, informed individuals. While an official government stenographer leaned forward to hear and transcribe every word, a staff member briefed the government's advisers on a subject that had been selected as an example of a serious problem requiring their counsel.

The subject, he told them, is called the artificial kidney—a small machine that looks and works something like a washing machine. This machine, the briefing officer continued, means the difference between life and death for thousands of Americans each year. It can keep alive individuals whose normal kidneys have been totally ruined with disease, by simply washing their blood free of the wastes their kidneys can't eliminate. An estimated 3,600 Americans—the advisers were told—come to require an artificial kidney each year. With the machine these people can continue to enjoy nearly normal lives. Without it they have no hope of living more than a few months.

Unfortunately, the advisers were informed, in the entire nation there were far from enough kidney machines to go around.

"We now have facilities to save approximately 100 each year," the briefing officer said. "And the other 3,500 are lost."

"There are 97 percent of these dying, as things stand now," he went on. "If they can't be hooked up to the washing machine and get a Jim Dandy job on their kidneys, they are gone."

The advisers were interested. They all asked questions. Was this the only way to save these people? How much did the machines cost? Was the federal government the only institution spending money to provide the machines?

Several pondered the great complexity of the problem. One asked about the difficulty of getting enough trained personnel to operate the machines. Another wondered whether it was appropriate for the government alone to pay for such a service. A third spoke about the unwillingness of Congress to spend more money to purchase kidney machines—or anything else, for that matter.

In the midst of this discussion someone wondered out loud about how to explain such a serious situation to the public. How could people be expected to understand why only one out of every 36 men, women, and children who need an artificial kidney can obtain one despite the fact that we have known how to build and operate these machines for nearly a decade? How could what the federal government was doing to remedy this huge need—or not doing, to be more precise—be adequately explained to an ever curious public?

"This is going to be a politically hot issue," another adviser agreed. How could a congressman, he asked, whose constituent was about to die for lack of a kidney machine, be expected to appreciate the many complexities of the problem?

A silence fell over the group. No one seemed to have an answer. Finally one adviser spoke up.

Problems like this, he began, should not be explained too clearly. They should not be outlined too explicitly for either congressmen or for the man in the street. In fact, he maintained, they should not be outlined at all.

"I would argue," he said, "that one of the subtle and essential parts of an administrator . . . is to blur issues. A clarification and sharpening of issues is not always desirable.

"I would blur this issue if at all possible," he concluded.

There was hardly a murmur of dissent. The other advisers seemed satisfied with their colleague's suggestion. They seemed in accord that no useful purpose would be served by sharpening this issue. Only one man, a government sociologist, seemed unhappy with the adviser's "solution." The decision about how many lives to save with kidney machines, he argued, could not be brushed aside so readily. The great cost of the machines in dollars, he said, was just an excuse used by administrators who wished to avoid thinking about the problem and coming to a decision.

"Why this?" he asked, making a motion as though slicing a hunk of money meant for kidney machines out of the federal budget. "Why not something else? Why not less of a price support on tobacco? Why not delay the moonshot a year? Why not build one less superhighway?"

He looked around the room, as though for a sign that someone agreed, or at least understood what he was trying to say. The minister's eye caught mine as the sociologist continued. Has anyone actually decided, he was saying, that people with kidney disease need perish for lack of some piece of machinery?

The room was silent again.

"It should not just happen by default," he said. "Someone making the decision, 'Well, that is a piece of money which, if we snatch out of the budget this year will take care of us, will bring us down underneath some sort of ceiling that we have to operate within.'"

I was beginning to see what the minister had meant when he said that the length of life was a social policy decision. Actually he might just as well have said a "non-decision," since no one seemed willing to acknowledge, in reply to the sociologist, that any decision was actually being made. No one seemed willing to admit that any course of action—or non-action—was being taken, even by default.

Shortly thereafter, the meeting was adjourned. As I left the room, the words of the government adviser—a tall, distinguished-looking man—ran in my ears: *I would blur this issue if at all possible.*

Surely, I thought, there must be a more sensible and palatable way of making decisions than this, especially decisions affecting the everyday lives of thousands of Americans. How, I also wondered, can one hope to blur an issue that seemed so vivid and urgent? The press and most citizens, I felt sure, would certainly see through any attempt by the government to cover up its failure to supply enough kidney machines.

My work took me into other areas and for a time I forgot about the kidney machines and what had happened at the meeting. Then, one day, I found myself wondering what the outcome of the whole business had been. I walked into the minister's office.

"Oh," he said. "They did just what they said they would. They blurred the whole thing."

"How?" I was amazed. "Wasn't there a lot of pressure from Congress and the newspapers for something to be done?"

He went to his bookcase where such works as Augustine's

*Confessions* and the *Five Year Program and Financial Plan of HEW* stood incongruously side by side. He took out two thick reports.

"There are both discussions of the artificial kidney problem. One was written by HEW, the other by the Bureau of the Budget. Both used essentially the same basic facts—how many people die, how much the machines cost, and so forth. One report concludes that a massive effort should be made almost immediately to supply kidney machines for everyone who needs them. The other report proposes a much smaller effort, only slightly greater than the one that was made this year."

"Both reports," he went on, "were written by eminent experts. In fact some of the same people served as consultants for both of them."

He shrugged his shoulders. "A press conference was held. Unfortunately, the reports were so long and detailed that nobody had really read them completely. Most people, congressmen too, threw up their hands in despair. After all, if the experts couldn't agree on what ought to be done, how could an ordinary person hope to decide?

"That's where the whole thing is now," he said.

In the weeks and months that followed, from time to time, I heard more about the kidney machines.

"You know what I spend most of my time doing every day?" a young angular-faced fellow, one of the administrators of the kidney program, asked me.

"I spend it answering letters. They come addressed to the White House or the President. They say things like, 'My wife died today of kidney disease because she couldn't get an artificial kidney machine.' That's what they say."

He smiled and brushed his sandy hair out of his eyes. "How would you like a job like that?"

"How do you answer them?" I asked genuinely interested.

"Oh, I usually start by telling them that the President has asked me to reply to their letter. I tell them how sorry I am about their recent loss. I say that, as they know, the artificial kidney is still in the experimental stages, but that we hope soon to be able to supply them for all who need them. Then I wind up by telling them that we sincerely appreciate their letter and would welcome any further suggestions they might have."

He smiled again and then, in an instant, his long face became deadly serious.

"You know," he said, leaning close to me and wetting my face as he spit the words, "I sometimes wish those bastards who make up these five-year financial plans, who juggle the budget figures each year, those pricks over at the Budget Bureau who set the ceilings—I wish they all had to answer a few of these letters. Maybe then they'd see things differently."

"What about the congressmen who sit on the Appropriations Committees?"

"They're different. If they had their way we'd have a national program right now. They know what's going on—they have people in their districts dying every day.

"It's the others. The ones who sit on the Budget Committee and can't make up their minds how to get the department under the Budget Bureau's ceiling, so they slice an extra million out of our program. Those are the ones I'd like to see answer a few letters now and then."

I was fascinated. He was speaking about a world I knew absolutely nothing about—a world of budget cycles, legislative proposals, administrative decisions—in short a world of government operations that was a total mystery to me. Very little in my own background seemed relevant to this world. My only contact with economics, an elementary course at college, had little relevance to the intricacies of the federal budget. My only knowledge of how the government worked was a vague remembrance of my high school civics course. It seemed clear that there was a lot more involved in making a decision to supply more kidney machines than was immediately apparent.

I thought for a long time about what this young administrator had said. Everyone, I imagined, who runs a program in Washington—whether it be one to provide kidney machines or to build low-income housing or to land on the moon—all must be men committed to their programs. All administrators must be convinced that their particular program should have more money. All must have persuasive arguments why Congress should give them more funds.

While I was in Washington, the Department of Health, Education and Welfare tried an experiment. All the HEW administrators were asked to estimate how much money their programs could use over the next five years, if they could have any amount. Needless to say, the total was several billions of dollars above what HEW was then spending or expecting to spend in the near future.

One day I ran into the sociologist who had spoken at the kidney machine meeting. I asked him about this dilemma.

"How could we get along without some sort of budget—without someone whose job it is to make sure the programs operate within some sort of ceiling? Otherwise the sky would be the limit. We'd never have enough money or resources to satisfy everyone."

"Look," he said, waving a finger at me, "I'm not saying every administrator should have all the money or resources he wants. God knows, there's plenty of waste in our programs right now. I'm not even saying that we shouldn't spend more to put a man on the moon than we do to keep people alive, or teach kids to read, or anything else."

He tamped his pipe and lit it.

"I'm not arguing with these priorities. Maybe we shouldn't buy kidney machines for everyone. Maybe there are a lot of other things that we should do instead. My argument is simply that it should not just happen. These are choices that shouldn't just be made by default, by somebody in the Budget Bureau looking at a graph which shows that such and such a program has been growing rapidly for the last few years and needs to be slowed down so that its growth looks more like that of the other programs.

"The reason that we aren't buying kidney machines for

everyone," he went on, "has nothing to do with the cost in dollars. None of our programs helps people to buy eyeglasses or hearing aids either—and these cost much less. They certainly aren't luxuries nowadays. Yet we know that there are lots of people who can't afford to buy them. No," he said, "the cost isn't the real hang-up. There are lots of things that cost much less that we aren't doing either. The point is that nobody is sitting down and actually sweating over these decisions. Nobody is asking how important it is to teach children to read or to buy them eyeglasses or to feed them a nutritious lunch. No one is asking whether it's more important to educate schoolchildren or to build more highways. No one is asking what are the gains and costs of each.

"I'm not saying there's any 'right' answer—it all depends on what people think is more important at the time. I'm just saying that, right now, we aren't even asking the questions, let alone coming up with answers. We're just letting these choices happen by default."

I felt as though I was getting in over my head. The whole business seemed so complex and insoluble that I almost hesitated to ask any more questions. The sociologist stood there patiently, as though waiting for me to say something.

"But to make the kinds of choices you're talking about," I said, "the nation—or at least the government—would need some sort of overall framework, sort of like an economic development plan, to put these things in perspective. Except it would be a social development plan. We'd need some sort of overall way of seeing how much effort we were spending on various activities, and where we might hope to make the most gains by spending more. Do you really think that kind of overall plan could be developed?"

"I don't know," he said. "All I know is that we have to try to develop a better way of making decisions about social problems. If we don't, we're going to come, more and more, to where the average American—in other words most of us—feels the whole system is too big for him. He reads about all these goodies like kidney machines or teaching machines, or job training, or school lunches, or what have you and he sees them on television, and then when he goes down with his wife who needs a kidney machine they tell him there's no room at the inn."

"One last question," I persisted. "Aren't federal programs always reviewed by advisory councils of experts to see just where the gaps are—whether we could be doing more than we are now?" Even as I spoke I thought about the advice rendered at the kidney machine meeting and the words turned sour in my mouth.

"There are lots of questions the experts can answer," he said, slowly, "but you'll find, if you stay in Washington long enough, that there are questions no expert knows the answers to because no one has ever tried to find the answers. There are no experts who can answer the kind of question I'm asking.

"That question," he said, knocking his pipe on his shoe, "is how do we get to the point where, for the things that people feel matter most, there's enough room for everyone at the inn?"

It was only a few weeks later that a headline in a Washington newspaper caught my eye. The government, it said, was about to halt what little financial support it had been providing for kidney machines. The article went virtually unnoticed. There was no outcry in Congress. No public officials protested. Most people seemed to pay no attention at all.

I thought about what the distinguished-looking adviser had said: *a clarification and sharpening of issues is not always desirable.* I thought about the government's reaction to the problem of supplying enough kidney machines. I wondered if this was the way difficult issues were dealt with by the bureaucracy, if this was the way difficult decisions were avoided or made by default.

The whole business had become so confused and muddled that it seemed impossible even to determine who the responsible officials or individuals were. Were they the men running the kidney program? Were they the budget examiners in the Budget Bureau or in HEW? Were they the "experts" who compiled the two contradictory reports or the advisers who participated in the meeting I had attended?

I found myself unable to sort out all the participants in this "decision-making process." But in terms of the final result one thing was eminently clear. The adviser's "solution" had come to pass. The issue, at least for the present, had been successfully blurred.

# CHAPTER
## 3

## *Seeing the "Big Picture"*

Whatever my official duties were to be in Washington, no one seemed in much of a hurry to tell me about them. It was only after about two weeks sitting in my small, prefabricated office, that I was summoned to see my superior, one of the department's chief administrators. He was a young man, about thirty-five, who looked tall enough to have been a college basketball player. The walls of his office were covered with charts and graphs. On one door hung a colorful cork dartboard. He shook my hand vigorously.

"I'm glad to hear you're going to be our new expert on child health," he said.

I started to demur, but he went on. The White House, I was told, had become very interested in the health problems of mothers, infants, and children.

Someone had informed President Johnson that the United States was the not so proud possessor of an infant death rate worse than those of a dozen other countries. In the middle of the night, the story went, the President had telephoned Surgeon General William Stewart and had ordered him to come up with ways of bettering our record. The result was an HEW task force. Its members were physicians, economists, sociologists, and government officials. I was to serve as a staff member for this group. Myself and some other "experts" were to undertake the job of finding out what could be done and at what cost.

"If you're not an expert now," the administrator was saying, "you will be—in about a week."

I accepted the task enthusiastically. Here, I thought, was something I knew at least something about, though hardly enough to qualify as an expert. During my year as an intern at the Boston City Hospital I'd seen plenty of the preventible illnesses that assail infants and children—especially poor infants and children. I'd seen infants with overgrown heads, or other crippling deformities, undetected until it was too late for anything to be done. I'd seen children permanently brain-damaged from lead poisoning or dying of tuberculosis or rat-bite fever.

As I thought about the year I'd just spent in that frustrating environment a host of experiences came to my mind. I remembered the appalling inadequacy of the City Hospital. "It's possible to get almost anything done properly here," I remembered one of my fellow interns telling me, "if you can do it yourself." Obtaining even the most rudimentary laboratory tests often involved persuading the technician, if he could be found, that they were needed. The hospital staff—nurses, supervisors, and others—looked upon the physicians as people merely passing through, much the same as patients, and therefore to be ignored as much as possible. The nursing students were nearly all white. Blacks had only the most menial jobs. There was an esprit de corps among employees that went far to promote cronyism and inefficiency.

I was not an expert but I was certain of one thing—the care of poor infants and children, and their mothers as well, could be vastly improved if only by designing better institutions than the Boston City Hospital. And I knew, or thought I knew, that the City Hospital was no better or worse at providing care than other municipal institutions that serve the poor.

I mentioned my belief to the administrator.

"You'll find," he replied, "that the Boston City Hospital is only a small part of the entire problem. You'll have to get used to dealing, not in terms of specific details, but in terms of generalities. It won't take long," he was saying, "to see the big picture."

I agreed with him. This would be, I thought, an opportunity to try to solve some of the problems I had felt so helpless in solving the year before. This would be a chance to try to deal with these problems in a less hectic atmosphere and in a more deliberate way. As the administrator continued speaking, I recalled the incredible frenzy of the year I'd just spent —a frenzy that seemed light-years away from this peaceful office where the greatest disturbance was the occasional buzz of the intercom.

While he spoke, I recalled an episode that had taken place only a few days before I'd left for Washington. It was not uncommon for a single physician to see fifty children in one evening on the emergency floor at the City Hospital, trying to render whatever haphazard care he could for the most seriously ill, and letting the rest wait until he could see them. On just such a night, a young well-dressed man pushed his way to the front of the long waiting line, holding a cute blond boy in his arms.

"He's got a fever. I have to see a doctor right away."

"I'm the only doctor," I told him, "and unless he's any sicker than all these other children, he'll have to wait his turn."

The man was shocked. His round face became livid. He was about to say something when the nurse on duty interrupted.

"His wife used to work here, Doctor."

"I'm sorry," I replied. "The child is no sicker than many of these others. He'll have to wait his turn."

The fellow's mouth dropped as he looked at the "others," all of whom were black, and many of whom had been waiting for several hours. The thought of wedging himself between these "others" on the hard, wooden bench must have repelled him more than his concern for his son.

"You wait," he screamed at me as he stalked out. "I'm going to report you to the superintendent."

After he had gone the nurse turned to me. "You don't understand, Doctor," she said sympathetically. "We take care of our own here."

Now that I had come to Washington, I remember thinking, perhaps there might be something I could do to counteract this sort of favoritism that often prevented the poor from receiving other than first-class care.

The administrator was ushering me out of his office. "Our finished report is due on the secretary's desk in late September," he was saying. "The ball's in our court, and I'm counting on you and the others to do something with it."

I thought, in the succeeding days, of what I'd been told. I tried to think in "generalities," in terms of the "big picture." I did my best to forget my experiences at the Boston City Hospital and to totally eradicate from my mind all the incidents of the year before. They were not really relevant, I thought, to what I now had to do. They were merely vivid episodes and impressions that must be pushed aside, I believed, if the whole problem of how to get better health care to infants and children was to be tackled unemotionally and effectively.

I tried to forget all the horrors I had seen: the pregnant women waiting for hours in crowded clinics; the children sent from school because they were behavior problems, when in reality they were hungry, or deaf, or had trouble seeing; the infants who appeared on the emergency floor with rodent-gnawed fingers or with the nearly invisible puncture wounds rodents made. I tried to forget the infant who died one evening because there was insufficient heat in the operating room, or the Puerto Rican boy who perished because a certain inexpensive piece of equipment needed to keep him breathing could not be located in time.

Over the next few days I did my best to study the problem of child health as objectively as possible. As a first step I tried to get an idea of how many deaths and handicaps in infants or children it might be possible to prevent through better health care. I started with the problem of infant deaths. I began, as any sensible person might, by asking other "experts" for evidence that better health care could save infant lives. These experts, both in and outside the Government, were optimistic. Thirty percent of all yearly infant deaths, one told me, could be prevented by simply reaching more pregnant women with health care. Another said 20 percent.

Unfortunately, I soon realized as I searched further, that these expert estimates were actually not estimates at all. They were really "guesstimates"—guesses based not upon any actual experience, but on personal opinion alone. I spent hours in the library searching in books and journals for actual projects that had set out to prevent infant death or childhood handicaps. I telephoned dozens of individuals all over the country. The results were monotonously discouraging. I was unable to find any program or project that had tried to prevent infant deaths and had objectively measured its success.

Everyone, on the other hand, seemed familiar with the size of the problem. It had been, so to speak, studied to death. I found dozens of government reports on infant deaths in every region of the nation—reports of counties in Mississippi with infant death rates as high as those in several "underdeveloped" countries. There were reports showing that black infants, or poor infants, or Indian infants have twice as much risk of dying as "others." Some cities had carried out studies that showed in exactly which census tracts infant death rates were highest.

By the time I'd been in Washington a month, my small office was piled high with thick treatises that described in meticulous detail the extent to which infant deaths were related to such factors as social class, family income, the height of a baby's mother, or the occupation of his father. But I was still unable to find any reports of projects aimed at trying to discover how much the problem could be ameliorated. I was unable to find anyone who had tried to see how much of a dent could be made by one or another method.

At first I was incredulous. I didn't believe my own researches. There must be, I thought, a great body of investigation I had overlooked. I knew that the government had financed a network of experimental infant-child health centers across the country. One day I ran into the director of one of these "demonstration" projects at a conference.

"Oh yes," he said casually. "Our Maternal and Infant Care project has decreased deaths in infants of the pregnant women who come to our clinic by over 30 percent."

I was astounded. "Why," I asked, "haven't you told anyone in Washington about this?"

"No one ever asked," he replied. "We do file a progress report every six months," he added.

That same day I telephoned the official in charge of special projects for the Children's Bureau, which had financed the project.

"Yes," he told me. "We keep all the reports from our demonstration projects for several years. I can't imagine anything in them that would interest you, but I'll send them over."

The reports arrived the following day. I skimmed the one submitted by the director to whom I'd spoken. The report contained a great deal of information about the experimental or demonstration project. It described how many people were employed, how many hours a week they worked, and what their professional qualifications were. It described how many patients were seen each week and what sort of services they received.

But the report said nothing about how successful the project had been in reducing infant deaths. It did not say, for instance, that there were fewer deaths among infants born to mothers who had received care during pregnancy after the project was started than there had been before. I was able to learn that, in the low-income Chicago neighborhood served by the project, infant deaths were 60 percent less than in other similar low-income neighborhoods. But there was no evidence in the progress report that this lower death rate was due to the government's new experiment.

I rummaged through a few other reports and found a similar story. There was no proof that any of these experimental projects were, indeed, helping to prevent infant deaths or to improve health in any way. In some cases, there were fewer infant deaths in the neighborhood served by the projects, but whether this was a coincidence, or had something to do with the government's efforts was hardly clear.

I telephoned several project directors. Each one assured me that his particular project was, indeed, "working"—that it was preventing both deaths and disabilities in infants and children. Many even had crude statistics to support their claims. But all the directors admitted that they were far from satisfied with what they were learning from their experience. All said that they thought that virtually no effort was being spent to learn anything about how well the projects were working, or how their operation might be improved.

"We have plenty of data on our families," one said, "but it's all in raw form, in computer print-outs. I don't even have anyone I can use to analyze it."

The maternal and child health program was at that time about four years old. It was thought of, in the government, as a highly successful demonstration program. It managed to spend all its funds each year. Its projects were run by universities whose reputations were beyond reproach and the program had had no scandals linked to it. Yet at that time, several years after the program had begun, Washington had no way of knowing how well its various projects were working to improve the health of mothers, infants, and children. Washington officials, moreover, did not even have a plan for finding out. Some money had been given to a professor at still another reputable university to develop such a plan—but this plan had never been put into operation. There was, in other words, no way of determining what, if anything, the program was "demonstrating" possible in the way of improving health or health care.

I spoke to Dr. Arthur Lesser, an official responsible for running the child health program. I asked him why more effort was not being made to learn how successful the program was. Why, I asked, couldn't we learn from the program exactly how much it costs to supply certain types of health care? Why couldn't we try to find out how many deaths or handicaps are being prevented by this care?

This official looked at me with a puzzled expression, as though totally surprised that anyone would want to know the answers to questions such as these.

"That can't be done," he said. "To collect that kind of information would require an extra clerk in every child health center. It's impossible."

The method of running the child health program, I found after working in the Department of Health, Education and Welfare a short time, was the rule—not the exception. The department had almost no idea how well most of its other social programs were working. No effort had ever been made to evaluate the success of these programs in accomplishing whatever social purpose they had been designed to accomplish. Health officials had no idea if their health programs were really making anyone healthier. Education officials didn't know if their programs were improving the ability of schoolchildren to learn. The men who managed the juvenile delinquency program could not say whether or not it was preventing delinquency. Officials in charge of rehabilitation programs had no way of knowing whether these programs were improving individuals' ability to hold a job or to be self-sufficient.

In the Office of Education, for instance, no one seemed to have any idea how much better we could teach schoolchildren to read by giving them more intensive instruction, by putting them into smaller classrooms, or by doing anything else. In the Welfare Administration no one seemed to know how much juvenile delinquency could be prevented by better youth programs. In Health no one seemed to know how many aged people could be saved from nursing homes by better home care programs, or how much mental illness could be prevented by diminishing overcrowded housing.

The plain fact was that very few people had ever really tried to find the answers to these sorts of questions. In fact, these questions were practically never asked by most experts. Perhaps they were considered too practical or unscientific. At any rate, for most problems with which government programs were concerned the number of people who had tried to show how much they could be altered—and who had evaluated their results—could be counted on the fingers of one hand. Yet for each of these problems there was a veritable deluge of "studies" that showed how large the problem was. There were dozens of studies relating each of these problems to race, income, family size, the number of years of schooling attained by someone's grandmother, and so forth.

The problem of infant deaths was the rule—not the exception.

"Generally," one former HEW official, Joseph Wholey, reported to a congressional committee after having spent several years trying to discover how well HEW's various social programs were working, "the federal government has made no real attempt to evaluate the effectiveness of its social programs or of local projects within these programs. . . . Often," he continued, " 'evaluation' has meant only . . . the preparation of self-justifying progress reports."

Another official, after conducting a review of all the government's educational programs and projects within these programs, came to the discouraging conclusion that "an almost unbelievably small amount of resources has been allocated to . . . evaluation. . . . Consequently, an unfortunate and major gap exists between enthusiastic claims of benefits and concrete data to support measurable effects of the programs."

Without any evaluation of how well social programs were

working, officials or politicians could praise or pan any particular program without fear of contradiction. In 1967, for instance, someone noted that for the first time in several years infant deaths had diminished at a somewhat faster rate than in prior years. Federal officials were quick to take credit for the drop. The same official, Dr. Lesser, who had told me that it wasn't worth the trouble to employ an extra clerk in the child health centers, began to travel around the nation giving speeches about how his program was solving the problem of infant mortality. At the time, there was still no plan in operation for evaluating his program to see if, in fact, it had been successful.

The opposite phenomenon could also take place. In 1968 the Joint Economic Committee held hearings on urban employment problems. During these hearings Senator William Proxmire asserted that federal programs had been ineffective in improving Negro unemployment. The senator pointed out that at the time the Employment Act was passed, the Negro unemployment rate was 5.9 percent, as compared with the present rate of 7.4 percent.

"Now, this does not suggest to me," the senator concluded, "that since the Employment Act was put into effect that the opportunities for Negroes to work have improved—they have not—they have deteriorated." If, Senator Proxmire asserted, one purpose of the Employment Act was to improve job opportunities, the Act had not been effective.

The senator's contention that the Employment Act had failed in this regard was unprovable one way or the other. The effect of any federal program in fostering job opportunity had never really been evaluated. In fact, there was very little information, for the nation as a whole, from which to decide whether there was more or less job opportunity for Negroes—or for anyone else—than a decade ago. There was no way of knowing, in other words, whether a federal "experiment"—the Employment Act—now twenty-five years old, had had any effect on this aspect of the employment problem.

The federal government, I soon discovered, had in effect been supporting an infinite variety of ten- or twenty-year-old social experiments without any knowledge of how well these experiments had worked to improve the lives or the environments of individuals. The government, I learned, had never had any officials responsible for judging how well social programs were working. There were no staffs set up for this purpose. *Whatever evaluation was done was carried out by the same men who were operating the programs themselves.*

There were some officials who were convinced that many of HEW's programs were working even though there was little objective evidence to prove it. William Gorham, the first official charged with responsibility for evaluating the success of HEW's programs became convinced, for example, after an exhaustive review of projects to detect cancer, that these projects had been successful.

"If we added so much money, we could save so many lives with virtually no question about it," Mr. Gorham testified before the Joint Economic Committee, after a review of many project reports such as those I had dredged from HEW's files.

No official could have ever made such a statement before— and been able to back it up—because no evaluation of these programs had ever been undertaken. For most programs, other than those for which Mr. Gorham and his staff had sought to evaluate, it was impossible to say what their effects had been. The officials responsible for running HEW's social programs did not seem to think it important to try to learn anything about how well these programs were working.

In my searches to discover how many children could be saved by better health care I came across an interesting document. It was an 850-page book that told—for every United States county—how many infants had died each year, for the past several years. I asked the statistician who had compiled this momentous tome, an elderly soft-spoken lady, what I thought was an obvious question.

"How many counties have higher death rates this year than last?"

Her brow wrinkled as she looked at me.

"I don't know," she replied. "I never thought to look at the data that way."

I asked her if she could undertake to find out the answer for me. Several weeks passed and I received no reply. One day I called her and asked whether she had ever been able to assemble the information.

"Oh," she said, "we finished tabulating that a few weeks ago."

"Why haven't you sent me a copy of the results?"

"I didn't think," she replied, "that anyone up there in the secretary's office would be interested. They never have before."

I could scarcely help but be puzzled by her attitude. Information existed that pinpointed, in a precise way, the geographical places where one of our most important health problems was most serious. Yet the person compiling this information obviously didn't believe that anyone besides herself would be interested. It had never even occurred to her to delve into her statistics even to see in which locales the problem was getting worse.

I mentioned the incident to a woman co-worker.

"Oh," she said, "don't bother old Evelyn. She's already overworked enough as it is. Besides, she's the only one who knows what's going on in that office. Without her the whole statistical operation would collapse."

Her answer puzzled me. I wondered whether the "statistical operation" was some peculiar entity that had to be preserved for the sake of prestige or perhaps in order to publish elegant statistical studies that officials could point to with pride. I wondered what good it did to collect piles of statistical data that showed where infants were dying each year if no one ever used this information to try to ameliorate the situation. Yet I had the feeling that this was exactly what was happening. As far as I could determine, none of the officials who ran the government's child health program made any use whatsoever of this data. During my search for facts on child health, for instance, I met only one official who knew which United States county had the worst infant death rate. None of the others had any idea or even seemed to think this information might be useful in any way other than to publish government reports about the problem. Perhaps the elderly statistician was correct. Perhaps none of the officials were interested in knowing precisely where the problem was the worst or was getting worse.

Washington, I discovered soon after my arrival, has an expert for nearly everything.

There are experts who know exactly what you earn every day. They know how much you spend, how much you weigh, or how often you are out of work. There are experts who know how many words your seven-year-old can spell or whether or not he knows where Ethiopia is. There are experts who know what you will be earning in ten years if present trends continue. They know what you can be expected to pay for a new house or a four-room apartment. They even know what the price of lipstick or stewed tomatoes is in your neighborhood.

There are special experts who can tell you all about yourself, if you are an American Indian, or an Eskimo, or black, or yellow, or poor. They can tell you, for instance, if you make less than $2,000 a year, just how many of your teeth need filling or when you last visited a dentist. Or how many years of high school you have completed. Or how bad the plumbing is in your tenement.

There are other specialists—much in demand—who can tell you all about the special problems of infants and children, or those of the aged, or of unwed mothers, or of high school dropouts, or of disabled veterans.

By simply getting together the right experts one should be able to find out about anyone in the country. By just getting the right men in the same room at the same time it's a safe bet that we could know all there is to know about blind teen-age Indians, or about pregnant, unwed Eskimos, or about any other sort of person you happen to be curious about.

It should make one sleep securely at night to know that there is a specialist in the government for everyone. No matter who you are or where you live, no matter your age, sex, race, income, socioeconomic status, marital status, ethnic status or any other status—somewhere in the government there is someone who knows statistically how well you should be doing.

Unfortunately, I found, the sociologist I had met soon after arriving in Washington had been correct. There were lots of questions these so-called experts couldn't answer. In fact, it often seemed that the government's experts were more concerned with collecting data than in answering any questions at all. Like the woman statistician to whom I'd spoken, when it came to a particular problem, it often seemed that the experts had simply "never thought to look at it that way."

The government's experts, for the most part, couldn't say where a particular problem was the worst, or was getting worse. They had very little idea what effect government programs were having upon a particular problem. Most of the experts with whom I came in contact were experts of what is, not of what could or might be. They were men and women who spent their lives studying what had already occurred. They could tell you what an average Mexican-American fruit picker can expect to earn this year, because they knew what he earned last year. Or they could tell you how many years of high school he can be expected to complete because they knew how far his older brothers and sisters had gone.

But there were lots of questions these experts couldn't answer. They couldn't say, for instance, how much more progress in school our fruit picker would make if he had a better school, a newer school, or perhaps just a smaller class or a more intensive reading program. They couldn't say how much more he would earn if he could also be enrolled in a job training program. They couldn't tell you how much better his health would be if his mother had seen a doctor early in pregnancy or if he could go to a clinic near his job.

The sociologist had been correct. There were lots of questions no expert seemed able to answer and these seemed to be the most crucial questions of all. Yet, the government was spending millions of dollars each year on programs and projects that were presumably designed to find out the answers to these same questions. The government's experimental projects, and in fact most government social programs, were designed on the assumption that a particular course of action would, in fact, result in better health, improved education, higher income, and so forth.

Do we really know how far our nation is falling short of its potential for bettering the lives of each of its citizens? Do we know how much better our health or education could be? Do we know what the capacity of our society for giving people fuller, more promising lives really is? Anyone who tries to find the answers to these questions is in for a surprise. Anyone who examines the government's social "experiments," who talks to the government's experts, who pores over their graphs and volumes of statistics can never think about these questions in the same way again. He can never have the same sublime confidence that somewhere some expert knows what could be improved or even what has been successful. He can never rest assured that someone knows in what city or county the problem is the worst, and is taking steps to remedy the situation. He can never even assume that most of our officials are taking new steps to learn more about any social problem.

Such a seeker after examples of unfulfilled national potential may be convinced from his own personal experience—as I was—that certain problems could be eliminated or at least greatly ameliorated. But even with a diligent search he will find little proof in the files of the government or anywhere else. What little suggestive evidence there is has been hidden away in unlikely places and is rarely brought to light. Nearly all our officials are totally unaware that it exists. Only someone who has a great deal of time and energy can ferret it out. Once he does, he may be convinced that there are lots of things that have been left half done. He may be convinced that for certain problems there is proof that it is well within our national capability to do a better job of ameliorating them by merely applying what some government project has already demonstrated to be possible. He may be convinced, as was Mr. Gorham, that additional funds would save additional lives from cancer. *But for most government programs he is only likely to be convinced that a great deal of time has been spent and very little has been learned.*

The group with which I worked as a staff member, was eventually able to estimate, after a great deal of persistence, how many more infants and children could be saved from death and disability than are now being saved. We were able to estimate, for instance, that if certain measures were undertaken, some 50,000 infant deaths could be avoided every year.

We wrote a detailed but concise report that was sent to the President. It was read by members of Congress. We thought we had done a good job of portraying the problem and convincing Congress that it could be solved.

Congress, we were pleased to find, seemed to agree. The lawmakers seemed to accept our conviction that a new child health effort was needed—and that more effort was needed to see how well our present child health program was working. Several new paragraphs were added to the Social Security Act in which our new program was described.

Each of us felt a certain pride in the Child Health Act of 1967, as that portion of the Social Security amendments with our program in it was called. We knew each of its several sections by heart: Section 505 that provided for a special effort for the early detection of diseases in children; Section 510 that provided for dental health projects for children; Section 512 that provided for the training of more people to work in child health projects; and finally Section 513 that earmarked money to find out how well our present child health program was working. The Child Health Act, we felt, was our own law. We had written it. Without us it would never have existed.

When the Child Health Act was passed, everyone in our working group was elated. Congress, usually highly skeptical of any new proposals, had adopted those suggested by our group almost as they had been written—proof, we felt, that the time we'd spent studying the problem had not been wasted. Congress, in a year when funds for most government programs were being cut back, had earmarked more than fifty million dollars for our new program. In addition, convinced that we needed to know more about how well our child health program was working, Congress had ordered that 1 percent of all money spent be used for this purpose. Our group had the feeling that, in a very real sense, we had accomplished something that would have a definite impact on the health of mothers, infants, and children in the United States.

Several months after the law had been passed I ran into one of the men who had taken part in the writing of the original report. I asked him how the new child health program was progressing.

"Things are just the same. There's been no change."

"But what about the new money Congress voted for preventive care? What about the new health centers that were to be built? What about the funds for evaluation?"

"Nothing's different," he assured me. The deputy director, he added, thought that everything was going fine just the way it was. "He even told Congress he didn't need any more money next year," he said.

I was flabbergasted. I knew the deputy director well. He was the same man who had complained that an extra clerk would be needed in each health center if better information on how well the centers were working was to be obtained. The deputy director, it seemed, already knew—in some extrasensory way—how well his program was working and he deemed it to be working sufficiently well that no new additions or changes were needed.

Joseph Wholey, a young Harvard-trained mathematician, served as co-chairman of the group that studied the government's efforts to improve infant and child health. Three years later he was forced to admit that all the study put in over those many months had been wasted. He was forced to admit that nothing had changed. As he put it, "Decisions taken on needed new thrusts in child health care became unstuck and were reversed over the next two years as policymakers came and went but federal program administrators . . . stayed on."

I was truly amazed at what had finally happened—amazed that one or two men, the administrators of the child health program, could thwart action decided upon by Congress. I was amazed that, in effect, a single man ensconced in the interstices of the bureaucracy, invisible and unaccountable to the public, could even thwart the possibility of learning anything more about the whole problem.

Here, I had imagined was an issue, unlike that of the kidney machines, that was clear. Everyone—or nearly everyone—was agreed on the general course that should be taken. Nobody wanted to "blur" the issue. One report, not two, had been written. Its conclusions had been agreed upon by everyone, including the administrators of the child health program. A new law had been passed and a reasonable sum of money set aside for a new child health effort. Yet nothing happened.

I realized, when the whole thing was over, that I had learned the difference between policy and action. Congress had clearly decided upon a policy—a course of action to follow for improving the health of infants and children— but no action had ever occurred. A decision had been made— but never implemented. The best ideas and intentions of many people had been, almost inexplicably, lost and forgotten. They had just disappeared. And worst of all, though nearly everyone who had participated in the making of the new policy realized that nothing had been accomplished, no one seemed to be able to do anything about it.

The child health issue had not been blurred. It had simply vanished. The momentum that had been aroused for doing something had been dissipated by the very officials who were responsible for carrying out the law passed by Congress. What's more, though everyone working for the government—and many members of Congress—knew that the new decisions had become "unstuck" nobody seemed to know how to make them adhere again. No one seemed to have any idea of how to get out of the impasse of inactivity that had developed.

I had experienced my first practical lesson in how the government reacts to—but does not necessarily act upon—social problems. The administrator to whom I'd first spoken, shortly after my arrival, had been right. There was more to the child health problem than the vivid details I had experienced at the Boston City Hospital. There was more involved in solving—or failing to solve—the problem than I had ever imagined. I had learned what the administrator meant when he'd spoken about dealing with the "big picture."

Yet when the whole episode was over and things were exactly the same as they had been before it started, I found myself wondering if the administrator had really been correct after all. Perhaps, I thought, it was not such a good idea to think only in terms of the big picture. Perhaps the "little picture"—all the unpleasant, vivid details I'd experienced—was not such a bad thing to keep in mind either. I found myself wondering if perhaps it would not be such a bad idea for some of the officials in charge of the child health program to spend a year or two at places like the City Hospital in hope that this sojourn might lend some sense of urgency to their attitude. Perhaps the professor who had spent more than three years developing an evaluation plan for the child health program would do well to experience some of the vivid details I had experienced.

Ultimately, in fact, I found myself seized with a strange, almost indescribable apprehension—not a fear that I would never be able to forget those detailed experiences I had had, but that they might gradually slip from my mind as they apparently had from the minds of the officials around me. I began to fear that those vivid reminders might gradually fade from my memory without my being aware of it, and that—as they did—a sense of urgency for doing something about the problems they symbolized might also recede.

It must require, I concluded, an almost superhuman effort on the part of the officials who think constantly of the "big picture" to also keep in mind the urgency of the "little picture." It must be nearly impossible for them to hear the distant sounds of the Boston City Hospital emergency floor, to stay attuned to the faraway, indistinct, unamplified voices of those who suffer there.

# CHAPTER

# 4

# *One Distant Expert's Voice*

In the spring of 1967 a man from a small town in Pennsylvania wrote a letter. He might have been a coal miner or perhaps a coal miner's son. He was nobody special. But he was fed up with second-class treatment. His wife had gone to a district hospital to have her baby. In the course of her delivery she hemorrhaged badly and needed blood. Unfortunately her blood type was rare and none was available. It had to be ordered from the Red Cross central blood bank. By the time it arrived she had lost her baby and had been lucky to survive herself.

When it was all over the man wrote to the Red Cross regional director. He wanted to know why his wife couldn't be supplied with the blood she needed in time.

The Red Cross official had no answer. But unlike most officials of large so-called public service agencies he didn't just write back a form letter. He could have answered the bitter husband by saying that the Red Cross does the best it can, that his wife's blood type is shared by only one in a thousand persons, or with a multitude of other excuses. Instead, for reasons best known to himself, he sent the man's letter—along with one of his own—to his congressman.

Once again, the whole matter might have been pushed aside. Fortunately, however, the man's congressman was not one to push things aside. Firstly, as the son of a coal miner himself, he was interested in his constituents—all of them. Secondly, as a member of one of the congressional committees that doles out money to the Department of Health, Education and Welfare, he was disturbed by the man's story. He may have wondered how we can deliver a pint of blood to a battlefield casualty anywhere in Vietnam within hours, but can't do the same thing—despite our thirteen-billion-dollar health budget—for someone in Pennsylvania.

The congressman wrote the surgeon general, chief of the nation's health services, and demanded an explanation. Less than a month later—rapid time for the bureaucracy—he had one. In fact, although the congressman may not have known it, his letter had set off an investigation of the entire United States' blood-banking industry.

Bureaucrats react in strange ways. We shall never know why, in response to the congressman's letter, the surgeon general decided to conduct an investigation. Perhaps it was because of the congressman's position as one of the keepers of the pursestrings. Perhaps it was that there had been other letters.

But this time, evidently, a pro forma reply was deemed inadequate. One of the surgeon general's aides telephoned me. He wanted, he said, a complete report on all aspects of the United States' blood situation. He supplied me with a list of persons whom I might contact in preparing the report.

"Put this one on the front burner," he said, without elaborating any further.

It didn't take me long to discover some of the dimensions of the problem. All over the nation, I found, there was a critical shortage of blood and blood products. What's more, this shortage was increasing each year as more people lived longer and more serious illnesses were treated. In many localities the need for blood outran the supply. Many cities had periodic crises when their blood banks ran out of blood.

But the growing need for blood was not the only aspect of the problem. Despite the scarcity of blood and the great need, thousands—if not millions—of pints were wasted each year. Thousands of pints, despite the critical demands, evidently spoiled on the shelf because of inefficiencies in the blood-banking business. "These critical demands," one Washington press release stated, "become more alarming when one considers the annual waste of blood . . . in 1965 this waste amounted to 1.8 million units . . . 28 percent of the total amount drawn annually."

This statement was released, several months before the Pennsylvania congressman's inquiry, to herald the birth of a new HEW program—the National Blood Program. I interviewed the director of this new program, Dr. James Stengle. He informed me that, although the government had the power to regulate virtually every blood bank in the nation, there had never been any standards set for how much wastage should be permitted. Apparently, the "alarming waste" had never been alarming enough for anyone to do anything about it. His program, he told me, was begun in an attempt to make the most efficient use of the "national blood resource." But, he went on, his was a scientific program, not a regulatory one. He described to me some "exciting" research being supported by the Blood Program to discover ways of preserving red blood cells for longer periods of time while they sat on the shelf. But it was not appropriate, he said, for the program to set standards to control waste.

For several years, I found, Congress had recognized the seriousness of the blood problem and had held hearings on it. Unfortunately these hearings were largely devoted to representatives of the various blood-banking organizations squabbling with one another. The so-called nonprofit community blood banks came to Washington each year to lobby in favor of exempting blood from the antitrust laws. "Blood," they said, "is not a commodity like gasoline. It is a living, breathing tissue." Others, including the federal government, opposed the blood bankers, saying that they were trying to exempt blood from the antitrust laws in order to be free to establish a monopoly and further raise the price of the already scarce substance.

Each year new hearings were held by Congress. Each year hundreds of pages of testimony were spewed forth by both sides. And each year the blood crisis got worse.

Congressmen interested in the blood problem were hopelessly confused by the dozens of agencies, including the Red Cross and its subsidiaries, that supply blood. Each seemed to operate with little or no relation to any of the others. What's more, each seemed to have its own standards of efficiency. A man living in Wilkes-Barre might pay twice as much for a pint of blood as someone living in Scranton, or vice versa. Processing charges for a pint of blood at Washington's Georgetown Hospital—the head of the Red Cross blood program told me—were twelve dollars. At another large hospital a few miles away, they were only six dollars. He could offer no explanation for the great difference.

The blood bankers seemed so busy squabbling with one another that they had little concern for anything else. I asked the Red Cross official if he knew exactly how much Red Cross blood spoiled on the shelf each year. He had no idea. What's more, his agency—the nation's largest supplier of blood—had no plans for trying to find out.

Year after year, despite thousands of pages of testimony, the questions that concerned many congressmen continued to go unanswered. Nobody seemed eager to testify on how to get blood to a small town in Pennsylvania more rapidly. None of the congressional witnesses ever spoke about how efficiently their blood banks operated or presented figures to prove it. None ever spoke about how quickly they could supply a unit of rare blood, or at what cost. None of the witnesses seemed to have any explanation for why a man living in the District of Columbia might pay more for a pint of blood than his neighbor across the Potomac River in Arlington, Virginia.

In all the pages of testimony these questions got virtually no attention at all from the blood bankers. Instead they expended a great deal of energy telling Congress what a precious substance blood was.

"Blood is life," enthused Mrs. Bernice Hemphill, head of one of the nation's largest independent blood banks, who thought that blood banks should be exempted from the antitrust laws.

"Blood is a living, human tissue," Dr. Rosser Mainwaring of the AMA agreed, as if this quality somehow made it less susceptible to price fixing.

My exploration of the blood business uncovered another somewhat disturbing fact. Practically nothing had been done in experimenting with new methods to collect and deliver blood. Again, the private blood-banking interests were too busy fighting among themselves to give the problem much attention. What's more, the situation in the federal government was no less chaotic. More than a dozen federal agencies had something to do with regulating the national blood supply—and none had more than the faintest idea what any of the others were doing.

The single government program that might have done something about the problem had done nothing, even though it had been established by Congress for this purpose. The National Blood Program was set up to try to solve the problem of delivering blood to people. "The staff of the National Blood Program," wrote an official responsible for the program, "is vitally interested . . . in seeking possible solutions to the problems of inadequate supply and inefficient utilization of the national blood resource."

One might assume, because of this vital interest, that the National Blood Program might have tried to do something about the incredible waste of blood. Unfortunately, for a full year after it began, the program had done nothing. In fact it was not until about three weeks after the congressman's inquiring letter to the surgeon general—who had ultimate responsibility for the Blood Program—that the program finally did release to the public some of its goals. Among them, the program's managers said they would:

> study the feasibility of a computerized national or regional daily shelf inventory system.

Evidently the program managers thought this inventory might help to eliminate some of the horrendous blood wastage. Indeed it might. In fact such an inventory system had *already* been proven feasible—two years before! As far back as 1965, Lockheed Missiles and Space Company had shown that they could make any blood-banking agency in the United States look about as efficient as a blind man hunting for anchovies in a supermarket. Lockheed had used a computer to keep track of different types of blood and to locate them instantly. In eight months Lockheed officials reported the pints of blood spoiling on the shelf had been cut in half by the new system.

Unfortunately the remainder of the story had a familiar ring. No use was made of Lockheed's methods despite the fact that they were published almost immediately. The nation's blood bankers paid little or no attention. Perhaps they saw no need for reducing the waste of blood by half. At any rate, the Lockheed discovery went into the bottom drawer, as far as the blood banks were concerned. And, to make matters worse, the National Blood Program was preparing to invest thousands of dollars to investigate the feasibility of something that had already been proven feasible two years earlier.

But there was another, more important reason the Blood Program had been ineffectual in dealing with the problem of getting blood to people who needed it. The program had been made the responsibility of the National Institutes of Health, HEW's research agency. James Shannon, the NIH director and the man with immediate responsibility for the National Blood Program, made it quite clear that he had no intention of getting his hands dirty in the blood-banking mess.

"In our judgment," wrote Shannon in a letter to Surgeon General Stewart, "the direct responsibility of NIH in this program ends with the development of the technology and the demonstration of its applicability of [sic] existing problems in the blood-banking field."

The Blood Program, in other words, would be happy to spend its time making blood cells live longer or studying the feasibility of using computers in blood banking, but as far as getting blood to people—that was someone else's unpleasant problem, despite the fact that Congress had expected, in setting up the Blood Program, that this would be its major concern. Unfortunately Congress had not reckoned with the possibility that James Shannon and his fellow scientists would prefer to keep their noses comfortably inside the membranes of blood cells rather than try to do anything about the chaotic blood situation.

One afternoon, I went to the Pentagon to speak to Shirley Fisk, the assistant secretary of defense in charge of health. Assistant Secretary Fisk was a tall, lean man with well-trimmed silver-blond hair. He sat behind an immense desk, a battery of telephones beside him. He told me that the Defense Department managed to supply our fighting forces in Vietnam with vast amounts of blood without depending upon any of the civilian supply. He told me about the Navy's development of a new process for freezing blood so that it could be instantly thawed and used anywhere in the world.

I, in turn, told Dr. Fisk that I saw no reason why the civilian use of blood shouldn't be as efficient as that of the military. I was convinced, I told him, that the feuding blood bankers should be brought together in some sort of national plan to improve the present muddled situation. I told him, with some confidence, how such a plan might be designed.

Dr. Fisk leaned back in his high-backed chair and peered over the tops of his sandy-rimmed eyeglasses at me. He shook his head kindly and smiled ever so slightly.

"You're young," he said, "and full of energy." He rose to usher me out. "I wish you luck."

Thus far in my foray into the blood business, I'd found lots of problems. But one thing still puzzled me. I could not understand why, a few days before, the surgeon general's aide had told me to complete my report so quickly. Why, I wondered, had he told me to "put this one on the front burner"?

The Middle East "weekend war" took Washington by surprise. The mood in the city was one of anxiety at the possibility that the conflict might escalate to involve the United States. There was talk of the President declaring a national emergency, if United States forces became involved. All attention was on the Pentagon's assessment of the situation and on the debate in Congress. At HEW, for the moment, everything else was forgotten. One official with an office near mine listened to the war reports on his transistor radio, an Israeli road map covering his desk.

During this crisis, something occurred to me. I recalled my conversations about blood with federal civil defense officials. I had not thought these interviews too important at the time. I had been bored with their descriptions of how many thousand bottles of plasma were stockpiled across the nation in the event of nuclear attack. But one thing stuck in my mind: in the event of a national emergency, there was supposed to be a plan for supplying blood—as well as all other essential emergency supplies—to all civilians. This plan was the responsibility of HEW. The Defense Department had the same responsibility for all military personnel.

What bothered me was that I could not recall anything from my conversations about this plan, except that it was supposed to exist. What official in HEW was to have the responsibility for running it? How were supplies, such as blood, to be shared between HEW and the Defense Department? The Defense Department, I knew, had contracts with all major suppliers of blood, such as the Red Cross. These contracts, in the event of a national emergency, would automatically be "activated." Did HEW, I wondered, have any similar contracts?

I spoke again by telephone with several officials. They were as confused as I was. One told me that, as far as he knew, there was no emergency plan for distributing civilian supplies. He did not even know who would have the responsibility for running one, he said. The surgeon general had assigned an aide to the Office of Emergency Planning, he went on, but this man had retired and had never been replaced. I asked him how long it would take to set up a national plan for supplying blood and other emergency supplies to civilians.

"If we had the people," he replied, "two weeks."

I remembered a newspaper headline I'd seen a short time before. "Viet Blood Use Rises 1,000 Percent," it had read. No official to whom I spoke seemed to know what would happen if the military's need for blood or other supplies kept increasing. No one seemed to know in what way, if any, civilians could be protected in the event of such further increases. HEW, one official told me, did not even have any funds that could be used for such a contingency.

I imagined, in contrast to this apparent confusion, Assistant Secretary Fisk calmly pushing one of the buttons beside his desk and "activating" the Defense Department's contracts with the major blood suppliers.

I was starting to understand why the aide had felt some urgency over the completion of my report. The surgeon general himself, I later learned, had sensed the "fuzziness" in the nation's emergency plans for blood. This, in fact, may have been his primary concern. It was probably the lack of any real emergency plan—and not the congressman's letter—that had led the surgeon general to ask for an urgent report on the blood situation.

I wrote my report and sent it to the surgeon general. The report, I thought, set forth the problems I'd encountered in a concise way. It mentioned the seeming lack of a national emergency plan. But by the time I'd submitted the report, events in the Middle East had cooled down. Washington became calm again. Talk of declaring a national emergency subsided. I heard nothing about whether or not my report had been acted upon or even read. The blood business seemed forgotten.

One morning, several days after I'd completed my report, I received an envelope in the HEW internal mail marked "for your information." Inside I found a copy of a reply from the surgeon general to the congressman who had written him. The reply was dated several days before my report had been finished. It "responded" to the congressman at length. It told him that the problem of blood wastage was really not so serious. It told him that the NIH was working hard to solve the problem. It told him of the plan to study the feasibility of using computers in blood banking. The reply, in fact, told the congressman a great deal—except whether or not his constituent in Pennsylvania would have any better luck getting blood the next time he needed it.

Inside the envelope was another piece of paper. It looked as though it had perhaps been sent to me by mistake. It was a copy of a note to the surgeon general from his assistant surgeon general. It had evidently been sent to him along with the letter that had been prepared for the congressman.

"This is just another in a series of congressional expressions on this subject," read the assistant surgeon general's note to his boss.

There had, then, been other letters. Perhaps even many others. And each of the letter writers had probably received a similar lengthy, but essentially "satisficing," reply. I began to understand what Assistant Secretary Fisk's enigmatic smile had meant when he had wished me "good luck." Suddenly I felt relatively confident I would hear little more about the blood situation.

Most students of government are populists at heart. They plead for greater citizen interest and participation in the affairs of government. They express confidence that—if the public will only make their problems heard—some action will ultimately result to alleviate them.

"The citizen who wants to wail," says Walter Gelhorn, "can be certain someone will hear him."

Bill Lederer, in *A Nation of Sheep*, urged ordinary people to write their congressmen in order to complain and press for change:

> No voice goes unnoticed, particularly if it is raised in intelligent question, objection, or praise. The unorganized civilian is potentially the greatest force of all.

Perhaps Gelhorn and Lederer are right. I can only say that, during my brief experience in the government, I found no evidence that this sort of letter-writing citizen interest had any effect whatsover on the way the government went about its business. Letters from citizens—and congressmen—were looked upon by officials merely as things that had to be answered, a necessary chore. No effort was made to cull from these thousands of expressions of discontent any ideas as to how the government might improve its programs. This vital source of "feedback" on how government programs were really working was looked upon merely as an unpleasant by-product of such programs.

The man in the street who complains to his government, perhaps through his congressman, will often receive a lengthy reply from a high-ranking official. Countless hours may be spent shuffling his letter back and forth between various government officials. In fact, the longer it takes him to receive an answer, the more certain he can be that it has traveled back and forth within the bureaucracy. The citizen who wails will indeed probably be heard. But will he be listened to?

What did the Pennsylvania man's letter ultimately accomplish? The discouraging answer is, very little. Even though it reached the highest rungs of the federal government, it resulted in virtually no corrective action being taken. Unfortunately the officials who read the letter didn't have the slightest idea what to do about the whole problem. Someone proposed a commission to look into it. Someone else proposed that an interagency committee, composed of specialists from various government agencies, be formed. Someone else suggested more research and planning grants to study various aspects more fully. A special report was prepared for the surgeon general, making him aware of the problem and making various recommendations. A letter was written to the inquiring congressman assuring him that progress was being made—the same way other congressman had been reassured before. But there was no commission or committee, or even a single consultant set to work to find basic solutions for the problem. There was no effort made to get the private blood bankers together to hammer out a plan for action. The officials did manage to decide who would be in charge of the blood supply situation in the event of a national emergency —but no plan was made for what would be done if such a situation ever occurred!

Now, at least, government officials cannot say they don't know that such a problem exists and just how serious it is. But it will take many more letters, it seems, before they finally do anything about it. By the time anyone reads these lines, the whole sorry business will probably have been forgotten, and our citizen in Pennsylvania will not have any better luck getting rare blood next year than last.

Of course one could always ask why the ordinary citizen should be listened to anyway? The answer is simple. The chances are, no matter who he is, he knows something the experts and the eminent men who devise and administer our government programs don't. He knows how these fine-sounding and infinitely complex programs affect—or fail to affect— him. He knows how they change—or don't change—his everyday life. He knows if they really are working. The man in Wilkes-Barre or Allentown is a distant expert in "Ultimate Impact"—what really happens at the end of the line. The federal bureaucrats may know how much money they give to Kentucky each year for schoolbooks. The Kentucky officials may know how much money they give to Calhoun

County. But somewhere in Peachbristle Forks, the tiniest town in Calhoun County, is an expert who knows full well whether or not his son's classroom received a new encyclopedia. And if it didn't, he probably has some fairly good ideas about why it didn't, maybe even some ideas the Office of Education hasn't heard yet.

Will the citizen who wails really be heard? He may be heard, but not often heeded. His complaints may even result in the writing of reports—but not often enough in action. His small distant voice will usually be lost and forgotten in the hubbub of government officials talking about the wonders of new technology and feasibility studies. His complaints will usually get answered in a way that provides no answer, in a way that tells him nothing about whether things will be any better next year than this. And his congressman, no matter how conscientious, will usually be too busy to do anything but accept an answer meant only to "satisfice."

Historically our nation has placed great emphasis on citizen participation in government. As the government has grown in size, however, the ordinary citizen's voice has grown fainter. It has been stifled by the plethora of commissions, advisory councils, committees, and other advisory bodies that have sprung up throughout the government. The "noise" generated by these groups, added to the usual confusion of government, have made the ordinary citizen's voice practically inaudible.

We need a way to assure that the real experts in "Ultimate Impact" get heard—and that their complaints or suggestions get action. If we cannot find this way, we will be forsaking one of our most powerful resources. We will be ignoring an important source of "feedback" on how our social programs are working to solve social problems.

Right now there is no such way. And none of the officials in Washington are looking for one.

# CHAPTER
## 5

## *Satisficing the Poor: The Story of the Poor People's Campaign*

During the time I was in Washington, the director of the Smithsonian Institution, S. Dillon Ripley, announced his intention to build a life-size model of a slum apartment in the capital's elegant museum.

"What an original idea," gushed Washington art patrons. "What a good way to teach children about the lives of the underprivileged."

Perhaps some of their enthusiasm was based on the hope that the model slum would enable Washington non-slum children to learn about "the others" without actually coming in contact with them. But, as Mr. Ripley grew more graphic, his patrons' enthusiasm began to wane. Mr. Ripley, it was said, wanted real smells in his model to show the stench of overcrowded housing. He wanted rodents and vermin—real ones—because there were real ones in the slums. I think, if he thought it possible, he would have wanted real people in all their real misery to complete the scene.

When I was living in Washington this model slum—like so many other social-minded projects—was still unfinished. But Washington had long since gotten its model slum, though not in exactly the way Mr. Ripley had planned. In the spring of 1968 the news spread that a delegation of America's poor were coming to petition their government. In the bureaucracy the reaction was one of total helplessness.

"What can we do for the poor," one official asked me, "that we aren't doing already? Congress won't give us any more money. Congress won't even give us any additional authority without money. Our hands are tied."

Everywhere the reaction was the same. In fact, many officials thought the poor people were unreasonable to march on Washington when the administration was having so much trouble. The President was battling Congress to try to avoid cutting the domestic budget. The lawmakers, led by Congressman Wilbur Mills, were pushing for massive cuts in spending in return for passing the President's tax increase. Everywhere in the agencies that "wage peace" the mood was one of despair. As the first mule-drawn wagons of the Poor People's Campaign rolled into the city, rumors were flying that more than a billion dollars would be taken from the HEW budget alone. Nothing, it was thought, could even be promised the poor with the slightest hope of being carried out. The poor, everyone predicted, were destined to go home empty-handed.

Most of the officials in Washington did not understand what the poor people wanted. Used to dealing with sophisticated lobbyists, they were expecting certain types of demands. Few of them, it is safe to say, anticipated the sorts of questions they would have to answer. And fewer still expected to face the sort of people who were to confront them.

The Poor People's Campaign came to Washington with all the cards stacked against it. The campaign had trouble getting started. It had trouble convincing ordinary poor people to uproot themselves and make the long trek to Washington. When they got there they found the mood in the capital tough. The city had been through its first riot. It had experienced its worst fire since the British sacking in the War of 1812. Congressmen, looking home to their districts, found little sympathy for the campaign. And government officials, as I have said, could see nothing they could do or even promise. Everything possible, they thought, was already being done.

When the campaign finally reached Washington, even the natural elements seemed to conspire against it. No sooner had the tired travelers begun to build their A-frame plywood huts near the Lincoln Memorial—on land nearly denied them at the last moment by Congress—then the rains began. Day after day the downpour continued until it seemed it would never stop. The encampment turned into a morass of slate-red mud. Even when the rains let up for a while it was nearly impossible to walk through the camp. One's feet were sucked into the red mud at each step. Shallow-looking puddles concealed great excavations that could send you up to your knees in water. At night the camp was pitch-black, except for a few lights, making walking even more treacherous. Many of the poor had no good shoes, let alone boots or galoshes.

It was like a scene from Dante. It must have been like being led through purgatory.

It must have been like being poor.

The builders of Resurrection City had done exactly what Dillon Ripley wanted to do. They had created a replica of a slum. Stores, a church, a hospital—everything was there—right down to the smells and the vermin. Their slum had all the ingredients of the real thing, including one that Mr. Ripley's would never have—real people.

And just as the Smithsonian's director had thought, other people *were* interested in viewing this new "exhibit." They came in droves. They came from the suburbs for miles around. They parked their cars near the Lincoln Memorial and sauntered up to peer over the wooden snow fence surrounding the camp. Commuters on their way to and from work slowed down to gawk at this model village. Washington merchants complained that tourists were no longer coming downtown.

The artists had done their work well. The camp contained most, if not all, of the miasmas that poverty spawns. The District of Columbia's health officer visited the camp and promptly pronounced it a serious health hazard. He tried to have it closed. Fortunately he was prevented from doing so by other officials who felt that poor sanitary conditions were an insufficient reason for preventing the poor from exercising their constitutional right to petition the government.

When the Poor People's Campaign reached Washington I had been working for the Department of Health, Education and Welfare almost two years. It had been two years since I'd left my job at the Boston City Hospital—two years since I'd had any close contact with poor people. Like most of the other young government workers, I supported the campaign's goals. But I had few illusions about what changes the poor could expect from Congress or the government agencies.

Despite the dire reports of goings on in the Resurrection City camp site, many young physicians—men and women—including myself, volunteered to provide emergency medical services at the camp. I remember spending one long night treating many of the same ills I'd dealt with on the emergency floor at the Boston City Hospital. But there was a difference. There was quiet resolution in these young men and women, most in their late teens and early twenties, that set them apart. There was a determination in them that was impressive. They knew they were unimportant—America's forgotten citizens: they had come to Washington to become, in some way, more than forgotten people.

They were well aware of the strange, almost desperate situation in which they had placed themselves. From inside the camp one could see mounted police encircling the site. They remained outside after dark at their peril.

"I'm worried about my girl," one boy told me. "She left the camp this morning and now it's dark. She doesn't know the city." He looked closely at me to see if I knew what he meant.

"God," he said, tears coming to his eyes, "she's only a poor nigger and she's lost. Can't you help me find her?" There was very little I could do to help him, just as there was little I could do about the medical problems I was called upon to treat other than offer rough-and-ready care.

The world inside the camp was as tough as that outside— as tough as life in any ghetto. One newspaper called the camp the repository of "rape, robbery and cuttings every day."

"I been on a lot of marches," a young girl told me as she sat on a stool in the temporary trailer set up for emergency medical care. "But the Reverend knows I'm leaving this one tomorrow. I'm afraid to go back to my tent. I know what'll happen to me if I do."

But, like poverty, Resurrection City wasn't all darkness, either. Most of the campaign's youths were not college-bred intellectuals, but neither were they totally unlike other, more "advantaged" young people. Walking through the camp at night one saw groups playing guitars and singing songs, much like a night in any other summer camp. Groups sat around discussing the goals of the Campaign or telling stories. Resurrection City, in other words, was a microcosm of the "other America," the poor person's America, with all of its faults and diversions, few as the latter may be.

It seems odd that so few people realized what Resurrection City's builders were trying to accomplish. It seems odd that the D.C. health officer could drive to work every day through Washington's real slums without a second look, but be so anxious to eradicate a mere imitation. It seems that neither he nor most congressmen and others who were shocked by the camp recognized its value as an accurate replica of poor America. The campaign's leaders had done exactly what the eminent director of the Smithsonian had planned to do—only they had done it in less time and with greater fidelity.

But the campaign had other objectives as well.

The poor had come to Washington to picket the government agencies. They had come to talk face-to-face with the bureaucrats, to rub elbows with the men who are entrusted with running the programs that run their lives—usually not very satisfactorily.

They came with a curiosity about this inept government that at times, verged on the comic. I remember one hulking black man who when he saw HEW's Secretary Cohen—all five feet six inches of him—said with surprise, "You mean to tell me that little cat's the secretary?"

But mostly the poor came in deep earnest. They were in Washington to convince the government that in large measure its programs had failed to improve their lives. The first day the campaign came to visit HEW, my phone rang.

"The assistant secretary wants to talk to you."

I went to his office.

"Look," he said. "I'm sorry to ask you to do this, but the secretary has asked each of us to send a representative to talk with the poor people. I realize you're busy, but could you spare a couple of hours? They're downstairs now."

I said I would.

"Why don't you go down right now. They're milling around in the auditorium waiting for our representative to come." There was a note of urgency in his voice.

I left his office. On either side of the corridor stood Capitol police. They towered over the rest of us. It was the first time I had ever seen police on the top floor of the department. They looked very ill at ease. Downstairs the scene was one of mass confusion. The auditorium was filled with people from the campaign. A scattering of HEW employees, most probably sent there for the same purpose as I, clustered in inconspicuous groups in corners. A man from the campaign was using the microphone at the front of the hall. He was urging his people to join in conversation with the officials.

"Sit on their laps," he said. "Maybe some of your soul power will rub off on them."

There were few encounters taking place, however. Many

of the poor sat in their seats singing songs and clapping their hands. I noticed one black boy, in his teens, who must have been raised on the Department of Agriculture's high-starch surplus food diet. He weighed probably 250 pounds. He sat there, dozing most of the time, occasionally waking and then falling asleep again. A man in a plaid shirt with suspenders was talking to an elderly woman from the Welfare Administration.

"You know how much I get to live on a month?" he asked her. She shook her head. "I get $56 a month. I get $4.50 a week for food allowance for each of us—my wife and three kids."

The elderly lady nodded again, but said nothing.

"I want to plant soybeans, but they won't let me."

I went around the room. Some of the poor recognized me from the short stint I had done as emergency physician at Resurrection City. They asked me what I was doing there. I told them, a bit uneasily, that I worked for the department.

"What do you do?" one Mexican-American boy asked persistently, but not with any anger. He sounded as though he might be interested in working there himself.

"I try to get the other officials to understand your point of view," I told him. Actually I felt momentarily ashamed that I had really done precious little to convey his point of view since I'd been at HEW. Many of the younger staff members pamphleteered and handed out leaflets on various occasions, but I had never participated in these activities, for reasons which I found hard to describe. For one, I had always felt uncomfortable about handing out leaflets to other HEW employees, and for another, I hoped I might have a greater effect in presenting "their point of view" through personal conversations with officials such as the assistant secretary, who might be able to do something to alter official policy.

Later that afternoon, when I had returned from the auditorium, the assistant secretary again called me into his office.

"I want you to help on the answers to these demands." He gave me a copy. "We've got about two weeks to formulate a reply that the secretary can live with."

The "Poor People's Demands"—as they were known in the bureaucracy—were like a final exam for the Johnson administration. It now seems strange, in the dying days of the administration, when it was eminently clear that Congress could hardly be convinced to take any action, that these demands were taken so seriously. Thousands of man-hours were spent in preparing replies to each of them. It was almost as though, in a last outpouring of energy, the men who manage our public programs were trying to explain all that they had been unable to accomplish.

Nearly everyone who had to prepare answers to these demands, even those unfavorably disposed toward the campaign, gradually admitted their reasonableness. Some even admitted, in private, that the demands were for actions that should have been taken long ago. The campaign had asked some tough and searching questions.

"They've really put their fingers on some soft spots in the system," one official told me.

What were some of the things the Poor People's Campaign demanded?

The poor wanted the government to take a second look— or a first one—at just exactly how well its ongoing programs were serving not only the poor, but also the American people in general. The Poor People's Campaign demanded for example, that the federal government find out more about what Americans were getting for their money spent on education. The campaign demanded, for instance, that the Department of Health, Education and Welfare increase the accountability of local schools

> by requiring that per pupil expenditures, dropout and
> survival rates and reading levels by school and grade
> be made available to the public. . . .

The poor demanded, in effect, that all Americans be told just how much their children are learning and how much is being spent to teach them. The poor people told the officials that they were fed up with the gobbledygook behind which the Office of Education's officials had hidden. That they were not to be fooled. That they knew full well that poor children in most instances did not even begin to get their fair share from the nation's schools. Don't give us any more gobbledygook, they said. Just tell us how much our children are learning. Tell us which schools are doing a good job or a bad job. Tell us in which school districts we—and the American taxpayers—are not getting our money's worth.

The poor demanded jobs. They wanted a chance to be trained and then work, especially in federal programs that are supposed to try to help them.

The poor demanded a voice in how government programs are planned. They wanted a say in planning those programs that are supposed to be for their benefit. They demanded representation on the councils that plan education and health programs, as well as welfare programs, and they demanded it at all levels of government, from the local to the national level.

The poor demanded courteous and dignified treatment from local officials who administer federally aided programs.

I read the Poor People's Demands at home that same night. Sitting in my Georgetown apartment I felt very far from the bustle of HEW's auditorium or from the darkness and terror of Resurrection City. I had never been poor. I'd never lived in a slum. What preparation did I have for interpreting these demands or answering them? Then my thoughts turned to the others—the assistant secretary, his assistants, and the rest. What did *they* understand about being poor? At least I had worked with the poor, talked with them, listened to their problems.

My feeling of inadequacy receded a bit, only to well up again as I read the demands of the poor for the immediate remedy of their problems. Each demand called forth in my mind a host of memories of events that had gone before, or plans that remained unfinished, gathering dust in HEW's files.

The poor demanded to know how well government programs were working. I remembered the meeting held that one afternoon to design an evaluation plan for HEW programs. What had ever happened to it? Did we know anything more about how well our programs were working now than six months ago? I was positive that virtually no one in our programs even knew for certain how many low-income people they were serving, let alone what was being done for them. When HEW had tried to evaluate its compensatory education program for poor children, there were only a handful of city school systems that could supply even the most rudimentary facts about how well the program was helping children learn to read or to do anything else.

I read the demand for more jobs. I thought immediately of the health industry—the nation's third largest employer. There had been a conference about providing more jobs for the poor in health occupations, I recalled, several weeks or even months ago. What had ever come of it? One thing I knew for certain—no government agency or private organization had pledged to provide a specific number of jobs for the poor by a specific date. As far as I knew the conference had ended, everyone had gone home, and things were right where they had always been.

The poor demanded some say in planning the programs that were supposed to be serving them. I remembered the paunchy man in the poplin suit who had come to visit HEW one day. He was from the FBI, he said. They were conducting what he called a "full field investigation" on someone who had been nominated for a position on an advisory council. The nominee was a woman and one of the few Mexican-Americans ever nominated for such a council. She was to be a representative of the poor on this advisory body.

"Why are you conducting this investigation?" I asked. "Isn't it extraordinary?"

"We do a full field on anyone nominated for high government position with recent foreign background," was the reply.

The government had literally thousands of advisory councils for the social programs that it administered. But there were precious few that even purported to include representatives of those very people toward which those programs were directed. Welfare advisory councils made no effort to include welfare recipients. Programs to aid migrant workers had no migrants on their advisory councils. Programs for the poor had no poor on their councils. The list could go on and on.

No information on just who these members were—except their names—had ever been collected. It didn't need to be. Anyone who sat in the council rooms of the federal government could supply the answers. The Poor People's Campaign knew the answers. The councils were not composed of ordinary citizens. Their members were not the poor, or the black, or the laborer—or even anyone who could remotely be said to represent these groups. Their members were "eminent" people—bank presidents, union chiefs, large corporation leaders. The same eminent people appeared on council after council. They sat for hours in well-paneled council rooms and deliberated, while their words were copied assiduously by government stenographers.

These councils were made up of the "helpers," not the "helped."

I could not help wondering if the woman under investigation by the FBI had been named MacIntyre instead of, let us say, Morales—and her parents from Scotland—whether her appointment would have been subjected to the same intensive scrutiny. I wondered how many investigations would be needed if the poor were to be given an adequate voice in the planning of government programs.

As I sat despondently in Georgetown that evening I wondered how anyone could ever hope to reply in a convincingly sincere way to demands that were obviously for actions that should have been taken long ago, for the redress of injustices that should have been corrected at some time in the far distant past. I was amazed at how accurately the Poor People's Demands pinpointed those things that I myself might have singled out as long overdue for change. In fact I could hardly help but feel somewhat ashamed that these demands—simply worded and to the point—had been assembled by the poor and not by the rest of us either in or outside the government. Perhaps the poor, not being in awe of the experts who design and run our federal programs, could more readily tell these same experts what needed to be done.

The Poor People's Campaign, unlike many Washington lobbies, did not simply ask for money. It did not simply demand some sort of special treatment, such as an oil depletion allowance or being paid not to plant crops. The campaign did not even ask, by and large, for new laws. The poor asked principally for something else. They asked for changes in the way officials did what they were already doing and had been doing for some time now, changes that would benefit not just the poor but all Americans. They asked that the government try to finish some things left undone for some time now, not just for the benefit of poor people, but for everyone.

The poor, it seemed to me, were also asking for a new attitude toward themselves from their government. This, more than a demand for new laws or new programs, seemed to be the real message of their campaign. One demand, above all others, seemed to stand as a symbol of the Poor People's Campaign. It was the most difficult to answer, possibly because it was the most important. It was the demand for which lack of remedy was least excusable.

The poor demanded to be treated with courtesy and dignity.

"We are human," one woman said passionately, during the meeting between the poor and the federal officials at which the poor had presented their demands. "We are not oxen." Person after person stood before federal officials and told example after example of disdainful treatment at the hands of those who were supposed to be trying to serve them in one way or another. In schools, in hospitals, in welfare agencies—everywhere the story was the same. Poor people were not being accorded the simple courtesy due one human from another.

This demand was taken so seriously by federal officials that it received an almost immediate response. The Commissioner of Education, Harold Howe, sent a letter to state officials asking that they take steps to remedy the situation. Other federal officials followed suit. It struck me as a sad thing that the government of a nation that boasts that all men are created equal had to remind state and local officials, like schoolchildren who had never properly learned their lessons, that all men were to be treated with equal respect—that even a poor man deserved to be called "Mister Jones" and not just "Jones" when he applied for food stamps or for Medicaid. It struck me as particularly sad that our government had to apologize for the way it had treated some of its citizens, but at least it was heartening to see how rapidly and affirmatively federal officials reacted to this situation.

Unfortunately the response to the other demands was less prompt and less positive. There was, in fact, a great deal of disagreement about how to respond to the other demands. Two schools of thought predominated. Some officials insisted that the poor be told about all the progress that had been made during recent years in their behalf. They needed to be reminded, these officials said, about how many new programs had been initiated, how many dollars were now being spent, how many new jobs had been created, and so forth. They should not assume that previous efforts in their behalf had been insignificant.

"We've got to tell them what we've already done. They can't just think this whole thing is starting from scratch," one official told me.

Others thought that the demands might best be answered in terms of what HEW could or would do in the future. The poor, they argued, were not interested in what had gone before. If HEW could do something, we should say so. If a new law was required from Congress, or more money, and

and our hands were tied, we should simply say so.

As more and more officials became involved in drafting the reply to the campaign's demands, there seemed to be fewer and fewer things that could be done in response to any particular demand. It was my job to speak to many officials and get their opinions on whether or not such and such a step could be taken. At every turn I found a host of reasons why nothing could be promised. For even the most insignificant innovation, there was someone who had a reason why it was not feasible.

The poor had asked, for instance, that they be allowed to share in the decisions about programs, such as Medicaid, that directly affected them. They asked that they be given a voice in the planning of these programs. Everyone involved in answering this demand agreed that it was fully justified. The only question, all agreed, was how to allow the poor their voice.

It was proposed that the department create a new advisory council, made up of poor people, to help advise on programs affecting the poor. New advisory councils, however, cost money to set up and run. It costs money to fly members to Washington from around the country. While nobody seemed to know exactly how much money would be required, the budget officers warned that they would most likely not be able to find enough funds. Furthermore the general counsel's office—HEW's legal arm—said that to increase the number of poor on presently existing advisory councils would require new laws, or a least new regulations. The officials who managed the programs said they could hardly compel states or localities to include representatives of the poor on advisory councils for their programs unless such representation were required by law. At present the most that could be done was to *urge* that the poor be represented, since some laws did require that some councils include "consumers." The definition of consumer, however, had always been left up to the states or localities themselves. More and more the roadblocks to greater participation by the poor multiplied.

By the end of May, three weeks after the poor had submitted their demands to HEW, those of us responsible for an answer had drafted nearly a dozen different documents. When the last draft was completed, I assembled all of them on my desk, in chronological order. I read the dates at the top of each draft, trying to recall the particular feeling I had had on each day during which we had worked on the reply: May 8, May 13, May 16, May 21, May 25 . . . As I read each draft, from first to final, I had the feeling of sinking deeper and deeper into the mire of bureaucratese.

The earliest draft, May 8, began:

> The poor are asking very simply, 'Find a way to eliminate poverty and deprivation in this nation and do it now.' This is our goal also.

The draft of May 16 began:

> My office and staff have carefully reviewed the . . . demands you placed before us on April 30. None of what you asked is unreasonable. There is no question about the fact that the country is not doing all that needs to be done . . . as you will see, I am immediately directing a number of actions that should be helpful. . . .

Still later, on May 21, the reply said:

> Together with my staff I have reviewed the . . . proposals which you left with us on April 30. . . . There is considerable validity in them. I want to give you my personal assurance that this Department will make an across-the-board effort to try to achieve certain critical goals which you have set before us. . . .

The final draft, on May 25, read:

> We have carefully reviewed all our programs and policies since we met with your representatives on April 30. Your recommendations and our responses must be viewed, we believe, in the light of the progress which

has occurred in recent years. . . . Within our available resources and statutory authority, we will take action to implement our responses to the fullest extent possible. Our responses are a summary of our objectives and proposals. We can amplify any points if this seems necessary or desirable. . . .

The early drafts were more detailed. They spoke of specific numbers of jobs to be created or specific time periods for actions to be completed. The later drafts were shorter. Virtually all the new or concrete ideas had been removed because someone had deemed them unfeasible. All that was usually promised—if anything was promised—was to "conduct a review" of this or that problem. Even then, no specific time period during which such a review would be completed was stated. The response to the demand for greater government participation by poor people, for instance, had shrunk to a meager two paragraphs. These paragraphs promised, simply, to "review present regulations and policy to insure that consumer representatives on . . . advisory councils are truly representative of the general public, including poor citizens."

Indeed the very way most of these "promises" were worded suggested a flurry of meetings, conferences, and memoranda rather than action. HEW promised, for example,

> to conduct a review . . . to determine the extent to which funds are being allocated to meet the educational needs of poor children.

and

> to initiate a program to review . . . whether minority groups have had full and fair opportunity to be represented . . . in key policy-making positions.

Reading the final draft of HEW's reply gave one the feeling of seeing an ice statue that had been gradually melted by the sun until only the vaguest outlines of the original remained. It was going to be difficult, I thought, reading these words, to convince the poor—or anyone else—that this was anything but the usual officialese that portends inaction. It was going to be hard to convince anyone, including those officials who were to carry out these "reviews," that these were promises that promised anything.

Perhaps the poor were lucky to get any reply at all. There were those who would have preferred that no response be given. There were some who thought that the demands were unreasonable or, in some strange way, that it was beyond the propriety of the government to respond to a ragtag group of blacks and Mexican-Americans. There were some who thought, despite the fact that many of the demands asked only for action guaranteed long ago by our laws, that the administration promised too much.

Several congressmen expressed the opinion that the demands of the poor were not really valid because they had not actually been written by the poor. In some cases, it was claimed, these demands had actually been written with the help of Federal officials. These congressmen took the position that any demands written by representatives of the poor were automatically suspect—if, indeed, the poor were entitled to any representatives at all. They took an attitude similar to that expressed by Congressman Rarick of Louisiana, after a group of welfare recipients had testified before his committee:

> I was quite amazed that they [the welfare clients] came into the hearing accompanied by a lawyer quite national in repute, whose office is on Park Avenue in New York. And their spokesman was well dressed, and he had the title of "Doctor."

"It would indicate," Rarick concluded, "that there are quite a few people who are preying upon the impoverished and unfortunate citizens in our country."

This attitude—that any representative of the poor or anyone offering them assistance automatically rendered their demands invalid—pervaded Congress. By this peculiar reasoning, not only were the demands of the poor invalid, but the government's reply invalid also. Senator Sam Ervin, incensed by even HEW's watered-down "promises" to the poor, sent a letter to the department. He wanted to know if the department had the legal authority to do all the things it had promised. The department responded by citing, chapter and verse, the various laws passed by Congress that gave it authority to do what it had said it would.

Local officials were even more antagonistic toward the poor and toward their demands. One local official lectured me for a half hour one day about the dangers involved in letting the poor participate in making decisions in programs that involved them.

"I don't understand," he concluded, "all this talk about giving the poor a say in planning government programs. Why, the reason they're poor is because they're poor planners."

The Poor People's Campaign, some said when it was all over, was a failure. It failed to offer, in Tom Kahn's words, "clear programmatic alternatives."

In a sense, the campaign was a bust. It ended in a whimper. Its leaders were unobtrusively jailed. Bulldozers and yellow caterpillars came and smoothed out the ditches and flattened the tents. They swept the camp site clean as a formica tabletop. The officials in bureaucracy breathed a sigh of relief. Washington went back to normal.

But did it?

Before they left Washington the poor people left their mark on our administrators and officials, even more so than Congress.

"When we first came to Washington," said the Reverend Abernathy at the campaign's end, "they told us 'We're doing all we can.' But then they found a few million here and there that they didn't know they had. . . ."

His followers laughed and cheered. But those of us who actually worked in the government knew that he was right. The Poor People's Campaign had taught the bureaucrats that they could do more than they were already doing for the nation's poor. And not just by discovering more money. The campaign had taught them that they could do more in other ways, too. For all its bureaucratic jargon, the government had responded to each and every demand. Even though very little of specific value was promised, officials did seem to grasp the fact that something could be done about the campaign's demands and that what was needed was not new laws, or even more money, but only the same programs, run perhaps in a somewhat different way. What was needed was perhaps a new look at old rules and regulations—and at the attitudes of those who formulated them.

The government could—and did—promise to train more poor people for jobs in its health, educational and other social development programs. The government agreed to hire more poor people for jobs they can do with little or no training, jobs in fact that they could do better than other people: jobs such as serving as interpreters for other poor people who can't speak English or being neighborhood aides in their own communities.

The poor demanded a voice in planning those programs that directly affect them. The government agreed to try to give them such a voice, to try to add more poor people and their representatives to the advisory councils that plan these programs.

The poor demanded a closer look at how well our public programs are actually working, The government could—and did—agree to look again at how well these programs were serving the poor—and everyone else.

The government reacted to the poor by carefully answering each of their demands. Unfortunately, as I had already learned, reaction and action are different things. Before I finally left Washington, I took out the manila folder that contained HEW's reply to the campaign's demands. I read it again. I asked myself what had been done since the final reply to the campaign to study the problems raised by the poor people's demands? Had even the reviews and reports, the promises to review "present regulations and policy" been completed?

As I read the department's reply I realized, though I was reluctant to admit it, that essentially nothing had been done. The promises made, for all their good intent, might just as well never have been made at all. The poor had been invited to choose representatives to meet with federal officials to discuss solutions to their demands. These meetings were obviously meant to enmesh them in the interminable morass of conferences and memoranda that are the hallmark of administrative inaction. The bureaucrats sensed, if they could only stall for time, that the poor would be forced to leave Washington and the impetus of the campaign would disintegrate.

Essentially nothing had been done after the initial flurry of meetings. The administrators had promised action but action—in their lexicon—was synonymous with an endless chain of conferences. Action meant an endless consideration of government regulations. HEW's lawyers, for instance, pondered long hours over whether or not it would be possible to better define the word "consumer" in the department's regulations so as to make it possible to put poor people on advisory councils. Action, to the officials, meant this sort of interminable Kafkaesque process in which, even if one regulation is changed, there is no guarantee that anything will be done differently.

About a year after the Poor People's Campaign, I ran into a young girl who had worked with me in writing HEW's reply to the demands of the poor. She had since left the department, as had I, but more recently.

"Whatever happened to all those reports and policy reviews," I asked her, "that were promised to the poor?" She shook her head.

"Before I left," she said, "one of my last jobs was to check up on all the things we promised the poor people. When I asked Mary Switzer, the welfare administrator, for her report, she denied she had ever been asked for one. She said she'd never received a request in writing.

"It took the health officials almost a year to even meet with the representatives of the poor," she told me, throwing up her hands in despair.

I showed her a list I had made of all the reports or "policy reviews" HEW had promised the poor. We went down the list to see which ones had been completed. Virtually none of the reports had been completed, let alone acted upon.

"Now you know," she said, "why I decided to leave."

By now probably no mark remains of the Poor People's Campaign on the bureaucracy other than stacks of official memoranda, and even these most likely have been swept from the desk tops the same way the bulldozers swept away Washington's "model" slum. There is little reason to believe that any of the promises to take a second look at how government programs work—or don't work—will ever be carried out after all. Or, to be more precise, there is little reason to believe that anything will be done *any faster* than it would have been done anyway. And that, as we have seen, is not very fast.

Perhaps, I thought—when the last of the campaign's mule-drawn wagons had left Washington—the poor people did not fail totally if at least they were able to make a few federal officials aware of the lumbering pace with which the government reacts to complaints concerning social problems. Perhaps the poor were able to convince a few officials—and a few other people—how slowly our government moves toward actually doing something about these problems. Interminably slow and meandering are the ways of the bureaucracy. Trying to make it act is like trying to turn over a long, sleeping crocodile by turning over the tip of its tail. This beast called the bureaucracy is adroit at reacting to annoyances from outside. It is masterful at satisficing its would-be antagonists by temporizing and promising future action. It is clever at co-opting its opponents. It reacts very similarly, whether the annoyance is a single citizen from Pennsylvania or a group of citizens from all over the nation.

The poor people learned all this about the habits of this great creature we call the government, but unfortunately they never learned how to alter these habits. Though the poor have continued to lobby in Washington, they have not yet been able to find out how to make the government act—not merely satisfice—in solving their problems. And unfortunately neither has anyone else.

# CHAPTER
# 6

## *The Famine That Fell Between the Cracks*

I can still remember the famous poster that used to hang in grade school classrooms depicting Franklin Delano Roosevelt and words from his "Four Freedoms" speech. One of the panels showed a young boy sitting before a table heaped high with food. He was gleefully spooning it away. That panel bore the caption "Freedom from want."

That poster hung in my schoolroom some twenty years ago. It may have hung in yours. Since then we have, doubtless, eradicated hunger in this land. Every year the Department of Agriculture informs us that Americans are eating better than ever before. For years now our most eminent professors have told us that our worst nutritional problem is not under-nutrition. Obesity, they have said, is our major menace.

Certainly the overwhelming evidence shows. . . .

Shows what?

One sunny spring morning a widely circulated science

newsletter crossed my desk in Washington. I glanced at it and the following words caught my eye:

Today, diseases due to malnutrition are rarities in the United States.

Unfortunately I had not time to read the entire article. I had to rush to Capitol Hill to hear HEW officials testify before a Senate subcommittee on the extent of hunger and malnutrition in the United States. The testimony told another story, a story not usually told so bluntly by federal officials. They told Congress that—although the true extent of serious hunger and malnutrition in America was unknown—the numbers of hungry or malnourished people *could run into the millions.*

The newsletter was still on my desk when I returned. I threw it away. It was worthless. Its editors and all the other experts were wrong. They were misinformed. The newsletter's eminent experts were writing about an America they'd been told about, or had read about, or perhaps had seen posters about. They were not writing about our nation in the year 1968.

Or in 1967.

One year before, Surgeon General William Stewart had been asked by Congress to describe the extent of hunger and malnutrition. Here was his answer:

We do not know the extent of malnutrition anywhere in the United States. . . . It hasn't been anybody's job. . . . We can do it all over the world, but not in the United States.

Even at that time, neither Surgeon General Stewart nor any other witness would dare deny the possibility that widespread hunger and even outright starvation might exist.

Other individuals testified at the same hearings in which the surgeon general participated that there *were* starving Americans. They had seen them. They had spoken to them and photographed them. They existed in many places—the

South, Alaska, our urban ghettos. These observers drew graphs, showed their photographs, and presented the results of laboratory tests. But they failed to convince most senators, officials, and professional experts.

"I would say that there is no starvation in New York," Senator Javits flatly asserted.

Archie Gray, Mississippi's chief health officer, was asked by Senator Robert Kennedy if he took issue with the statement that widespread malnutrition existed in his state. "Yes, absolutely," he replied.

"The amount we give public assistance recipients for food," Illinois' Welfare Director Harold Swank noted, "does not provide complete access to all of the items on the grocers' shelves," but, he asserted, recipients "should have access to essentials. . . ."

"If all this is true," said one southern official skeptically, "why don't we see more folks with starvation in our hospitals?"

Perhaps he wasn't looking hard enough. Less than a year later—in the privacy of their own homes—all Americans could see, in color, malnourished Americans both in and out of hospitals. It took a CBS television documentary to shake officials and lawmakers out of their ignorance with regard to hunger and malnutrition in this country. This documentary showed hungry and starving Americans in the affluent suburbs of our cities. It showed them in the midst of rich farmland. It showed them on an Indian reservation—the legal responsibility of the government.

Ironically this documentary was shown only days before congressional hearings were again scheduled—a year after the first hearings—on the subject of hunger and malnutrition.

I watched it with George Silver, the senior HEW official who was to testify at these hearings.

"What can you say," I asked him "beyond what every member of Congress hasn't seen for himself tonight?" He shook his head in silence.

At the time I had been assigned the job of gathering facts

on hunger and malnutrition for the government's testimony. The day preceding the CBS documentary, in fact, I had telephoned the director of HEW's Bureau of Indian Health.

"How many cases of outright malnutrition," I asked, "were seen in the government's Indian hospitals last year?"

"We don't keep any records in that detail," was the director's reply.

The day following the CBS documentary I thought about what I'd been told by the Indian health director. The documentary had spent considerable time depicting starvation on an Indian reservation. CBS had interviewed an HEW official at the Indian Hospital in Tuba City, Arizona. The more I thought about it, the more I felt certain that the director, or one of his subordinates, must know more about the situation in Tuba City than I'd been told.

The more I pondered, the more certain I became that the director had simply denied any knowledge of the situation in the hope that I would not persist in my inquiry. I was almost positive that he possessed information that he had withheld from me. Yet I could hardly accuse him of lying. He would simply deny the accusation, thereby dashing any chance of my obtaining whatever facts he did have. I had only one small advantage, namely, that the director did not have the slightest idea who I was. He only knew that I was working in the secretary's office.

I decided to try another approach. I resolved to try to take advantage of the director's ignorance of my own position or of what power I might wield.

I repeated my telephone call of the day before. The director again maintained his ignorance of the extent of malnutrition in Indian hospitals. He knew nothing, he said, about Tuba City, Arizona. I then pointed out to him, mustering as much authority in my voice as I could, that he had better find out exactly what the situation was. It would be embarrassing in the extreme, I pointed out, for Congress to learn that CBS knew more about the extent of malnutrition among Indians than he did. It might, I continued, even affect his image as a competent administrator with his Appropriations Committee.

"And that," I assured him, "will be exactly what Congress will discover unless you can produce some information on the extent of malnutrition in Indians by the close of business today. I shall see to it myself," I ended, without the slightest idea of how I would carry out my threat.

The information—such as it was—arrived on my desk that afternoon. It was delivered by special messenger and was marked "Administrative Confidential." From it I learned, among other things, that no less than eight children had been treated at the Tuba City hospital for kwashiorkor—a severe form of malnutrition—in the past ten months. Another forty-four patients were listed only as having malnutrition. Another thirteen infants, under one year of age, were said to have had marasmus—another type of malnutrition.

The CBS documentary had been correct after all. What's more, there was no telling how many starving Indian children existed in places other than Tuba City. Or, for that matter, how many starving American children. Or how many starving Americans.

Buried in the files of the bureaucracy was proof of a serious situation that no one had ever dreamed could exist. There was proof of a serious problem that subordinates had never brought to the attention of their superiors. It took a television documentary to make supposedly responsible officials disgorge what little information was available.

As further information was assembled from various parts of the nation, it became clear that malnutrition—among Indians, children, the aged, and the poor of all ages—was more than a possibility. George Silver's large office became cluttered with reports from all over the nation, not just from Indian reservations or from the Mississippi Delta. Children were found with advanced malnutrition in New York City, despite Senator Javits' assertion that such a thing was impossible. Other members of Congress found the same situation in their neighborhoods.

"I had a survey conducted in my state," said Rhode
Island's Claiborne Pell, "[to see] what the degree of malnutrition or hunger was ... the reports that I received ... indicated that in the last few years we have had 16 deaths attri-
buted to malnutrition."

Moreover there was good reason to believe that these reports of outright malnutrition revealed only the tip of a very
large iceberg. HEW's testimony before Congress put it this
way:

> there is strong reason for believing that a large pro-
> portion of those whose incomes fall below poverty
> levels ... may be underfed and undernourished.

This may not seem like a very startling statement until one
realizes that more than 20 million Americans have incomes
that "fall below poverty levels." Did HEW's testimony mean
that 10 million of them are undernourished? Did a "large
proportion" mean more than half? No one would hazard a
guess. Even Congress—usually quick to pounce on any statement by an official that sounds vague—was too terrified of
the answer to ask.

Some of the nation's top experts may have been too scared
to tell them. I asked one federal official what he would say
if a congressman *were* to ask just how many Americans were
starving.

"Too many," he replied laconically.

Just how profound was our aggregate ignorance of how
much hunger and malnutrition existed in America in 1968?

One of the first people to whom I spoke—in an attempt to
answer this question—was a lady nutritionist from the Agriculture Department. She was a personable woman with a
plump, ruddy face and a bright flower-print dress with what
looked like tubers on it. For years now, she said, the Agriculture Department had been making surveys of the dietary
habits of Americans. For years, these surveys had shown,
according to the department, that Americans were getting
a diet adequate in calories and proteins.

"What do these surveys really measure?" I asked this woman official at the Department of Agriculture. She told me a peculiar story.

"We measure," she said, "what food comes into the households. We ask the homemaker how much food of various sorts she bought that week. Then we estimate the nutritional content of this food. Then we divide it among the members of the household."

It would be hard, I could not help but think, to imagine a less precise way of measuring the nutrition of people. It seemed similar to someone trying to tell how well an automobile was put together by noting how much sheet steel, glass, and rubber were delivered to the factory each Monday. It almost seemed as though the department had tried to design a survey that could not answer anything—a survey that could not uncover the nutritional deficiencies of infants, children, pregnant women, or anyone else. Moreover, this was a survey that took for granted that—in her pride—a poor woman would not often lie about how little food she had been able to feed her family that week.

When the government finally did get around to looking in more detail at the problem that the Department of Agriculture had been "surveying" for years, the results were far from encouraging. George Silver, a deputy assistant secretary of HEW, testified before Congress on the preliminary results of these first more thorough studies. These studies, he said, "indicate that . . . preschool children show real differences in height as well as in certain chemical factors in the blood," depending upon their race and income.

"There is clear evidence," Dr. Silver concluded, "of inadequate food intake among poor children."

Numerous other, less extensive investigations confirmed Dr. Silver's conclusion. My discovery of a handful of truly starving Indian children was indeed only the discovery of the tip of an icebreg. Some 8 million people on welfare— the poorest of the poor—get inadequate diets, a government report estimated. A study of welfare recipients in Cook County, Illinois, where the welfare director had said that food allowances didn't let people buy all the items on grocer's shelves, only "essentials," uncovered some surprising facts. The amount of money allotted welfare clients for food, the study found, would not even let them buy the Welfare Department's recommended diet! What's more, this diet—if they had been able to purchase it—would not have supplied the minimal nutritional amounts recommended by the United States Agriculture Department. A "pilot study" of low-income preschool children found that the amount of protein in their blood was "consistently at the low limit of normal," suggesting that these children were receiving inadequate amounts of protein in their diets. Vitamin levels in the childrens' blood and urine were also low enough "to indicate limited recent intake of fresh fruits and vegetables."

Since no one had ever taken the trouble to determine, or even to estimate, how many people were inadequately fed, there was never any way to see if the Agriculture Department's food programs were helping alleviate the problem. Senator Robert Kennedy asked Surgeon General Stewart if there was any way to find out whether the food stamp program was adequate to alleviate dietary problems.

"At the present time," replied Stewart, "we have no way of knowing whether the program is actually alleviating malnutrition, because we have no base line." The same thing held true, he added, for the surplus food program.

The Department of Agriculture itself had made only the most feeble efforts to see what effect, if any, its massive food programs had had on hunger and malnutrition in the United States. One survey of children in Mississippi—carried out the same way as the national survey the woman nutritionist had described to me—tried to see if food programs had made any difference in the heights and weights of these children. This study, if it could be called a study, used height and weight standards set in the post-World War II era to judge children

in 1968. The results of the study—to make matters worse—
were that no effect of the food program upon these children
could be shown.

Dr. Silver told Congress that this study using even these
crude methods and outdated standards "suggests . . . that nutritional consumption may be no better, if not worse, at
present than in 1955."

"At the present time," testified Agriculture Secretary Freeman in June, 1968, "over two million children are being
reached with free and reduced-price lunches, but we estimate that at least two and possibly four million other equally
deserving children are not." The very vagueness of the secretary's estimate of how many poor children fail to get school
lunches was ample evidence of how much the Department
knew concerning the effect of its school nutrition program.

Bit by bit, HEW's estimate of the magnitude of the malnutrition problem began to seem less implausible. Some
people, however, were still not moved. "What we need is
fewer charges [sic] by amateurs . . ." replied an Illinois
official commenting on the report on welfare clients that had
been prepared by medical and law students. Other people
argued that the government's programs could hardly be
faulted for failing to provide people with enough to eat, since
this was never their intent.

"You understand very well," Senator Ellender, chairman of
the Senate Agriculture Committee, explained about the
school milk program, "that the special milk program was for
the producer, rather than a program to assist children . . . it
was done to get rid of enormous surpluses." The surplus
commodity program, Ellender also explained, was not a
program to nourish people. "We did not have in mind," he
said, with some degree of understatement, "the number of
calories we would give."

Senator Ellender's description of the food programs was
an understatement, indeed. The Agriculture Department fed
people whatever foods happened to be in surplus at the
moment, regardless of their nutritional needs or the nutri-

tional content of the foods. The government, in other words, was force-feeding thousands of people, much the same way geese are force-fed to produce pâté de foie gras. And it had been doing this for several years. Like the geese, it's probable that these people were getting a grossly unbalanced diet, since protein-rich foods were rarely in surplus. Yet officials persistently assumed that the range of surplus foods offered was quite adequate for a balanced diet.

"The current mix of commodities now available," said Secretary of Agriculture Freeman, "will provide on a daily basis—if used—almost 90 percent of the protein" needed in the diet.

Perhaps Secretary Freeman was correct. But his statement was only intended to reassure everyone that it was possible for poor people using surplus foods to obtain an adequate diet. Whether in fact they actually did or not, Mr. Freeman would not venture to say.

When Agriculture Department experts finally got around to looking at whether or not they did, however, they found some interesting—and disconcerting—things. When they studied the diets of low-income families being fed by the Agriculture Department's food programs they found, as an official told Congress, that "total caloric intake was at the low level of normal . . . the average diet was judged poor in about 60 percent of the families studied. Milk products, vegetables, and fruits were significantly lacking." The report of this study, furthermore, contained the following statement:

> The money value of the food used averaged $4 per person a week (including value of free food stamps and donated commodities). This is about $1.25 less than the cost of the USDA low-cost food plan for the South. Nutritionally adequate diets can be obtained for less than the cost of this food plan, but . . . families who spend less than this food plan requires are likely to have faulty diets.

Even this "study" was not really designed to find out

whether these families were undernourished. It was carried out in the same haphazard manner that previous federal diet studies had been done—by interviews and questionnaires. Outside the government, knowledge of the malnutrition problem was no better. The Citizen's Board of Inquiry into Hunger and Malnutrition in the United States, a private group, asked 75 food manufacturing companies the following: (a) What steps are being taken to determine the number of people now being excluded from the domestic food market because of low income, and (b) what remedial efforts were they engaged in. Here's what was found from the 35 companies that responded:

> We learned that there has been little activity in the private sector in determining the food needs of the poor. . . . Many of the responding companies referred us to the Nutrition Foundation which is supported by one of the leading food companies, and which sponsors research in universities and conducts nutrition education programs. This foundation was cited continually as a focus for private efforts. . . .

The Board of Inquiry then wrote to the Nutrition Foundation. Here is the reply they got:

> The eating habits and nutritional status of low-income families have been and are now being studied by both state and federal agencies. . . . The U.S. Department of Agriculture, the U.S. Public Health Service, the Children's Bureau . . . have been and are currently making rather extensive studies on the nutritional status of the low socioeconomic segment of the population and particularly in some of the southern states.

The board then searched for this seeming wealth of information and studies being done by "both state and federal agencies." Their conclusion was as follows:

> We have been unable to find such information or any such "extensive studies."

The reason was that no such information or studies existed. Private industry, the Nutrition Foundation, our universities, and several federal and state agencies—each assumed the others were doing something, while nothing was being done. For years the government and private industry had assumed—on the basis of "extensive studies" that did not exist —that nearly all Americans were eating adequate amounts of protein and vitamins. Nobody ever thought to question how thoroughly the problem was being studied. No one ever thought to ask whether the studies were really adequate to set our minds at ease. Our officials preferred to take the easy way out and to assume that, since they heard no commotion to the contrary, everything was all right. They chose, in other words, to ignore the possibility that any problem might exist.

Unfortunately this is not the end of this incredible story of social astigmatism—this failure to see an immense problem arising in the midst of national prosperity. It is possible, one might think, that our officials' ignorance of the problem of hunger and malnutrition was due merely to its great size and complexity. It must be, after all, a nearly impossible feat to determine the extent of hunger and malnutrition in the United States. It must be equally difficult to tell just how well such far-flung efforts as our food distribution programs are working. These are questions that could conceivably take years to answer accurately even if we had started years ago.

Oddly enough we did start years ago—but not in the United States. One day I was talking with HEW's chief nutrition expert, Dr. Arnold Schaefer. Congress had finally gotten around to ordering HEW to carry out a national nutrition survey. In the words of the original law, Congress had ordered the Department to

> make a comprehensive survey of the incidence and location of serious hunger and malnutrition and health problems incident thereto in the United States.

I asked Dr. Schaefer if conducting such a survey would pose any technical problems.

"Oh no," he replied. "We'll do it the same way we did our foreign surveys with the Defense Department."

Several years ago, he said, the departments of Defense and Health, Education and Welfare began to conduct nutrition surveys in some dozen foreign countries. These surveys were well conceived and well executed. They did what no survey in this country had ever done, namely, tell how well-nourished people actually are. In their zeal to study foreign lands, however, the government-supported researchers neglected their own. Dozens of grants were given out to study malnutrition in Africa or South and Central America, while the United States was passed over or more likely never even thought of. Meanwhile these same researchers kept saying that *our* problem was obesity and overnutrition.

"There is a group," Surgeon General Stewart told Congress, "very active in doing these surveys in other countries. . . . We intend . . . to use this skill and knowledge now to make these surveys on the domestic scene."

The government's experts were so certain, in fact, that only "underdeveloped" nations could have a malnutrition problem that they also went ahead and designed ways of combating the problem in every nation except our own. When Senator Claiborne Pell asked Agriculture Secretary Freeman whether protein-rich foods such as fish could be added to the list of foods distributed to low-income Americans, here is the response he got:

> FREEMAN: I don't think we could. It [fish protein] could be used under Public Law 480, but in . . . our domestic distribution program, it would not qualify as a farm surplus commodity at all.
> SENATOR PELL: Would any fish products be eligible under the farm surplus commodity program?
> FREEMAN: No.

What Secretary Freeman was telling Senator Pell is that

under Public Law 480—the foreign currency program—our government could supply fish protein to any nation in the world except our own. We could feed fish protein to starving Indians in Calcutta, but not to starving Indians in Arizona.

Fortunately, our seeming inability to devise ways of putting American know-how to work to assure an adequate diet for everyone finally began to outrage ordinary citizens. It outraged the men who made the trips through the South to document the presence of hunger and malnutrition for congressional committees. It outraged the men who made the CBS documentary. It outraged men like Robert Choate, an Arizona businessman and self-trained expert on malnutrition in the United States, who organized, with others, the Citizens' Board of Inquiry.

"We make better use of nutrition knowledge for pets than we do for the poor," said Mr. Choate about United States attempts to deal with nutrition problems.

Robert Choate is a good example of one man who refused to believe that there could be no malnutrition problem in the United States. For several years—often without any financial assistance but his own resources—he persisted in trying to prove that starvation could be a problem in America. He goaded administrators and officials to find out something about it. He stimulated Congress to hold hearings. Robert Choate is a good example of a single man—with will and perseverance—trying to get to the bottom of a problem that all our self-styled experts with academic degrees and professorships had chosen to ignore.

One afternoon Mr. Choate called me on the telephone. He was trying, he said, to identify those counties in the United States where the effects of hunger and malnutrition were worst. He asked if I had any information that might help.

On my desk were two computer print-outs. Both were several inches thick. Unfolded, they would probably have reached from HEW to the Capitol. They contained information on the exact number of infant deaths and premature infant births in every county in the United States, from

Autauga, Alabama, to Yellowstone National Park, Wyoming. Such information, I told Mr. Choate, was all the department had that might be of use to him. Unfortunately, I said, none of this data had ever been analyzed for patterns or trends. I had tried to get HEW's statistical bureau to do such an analysis, but they had told me no computer programmers were available, and nothing could be done.

"Doesn't malnutrition cause mothers to give birth to premature infants?" he asked. "Doesn't it cause death in infancy?"

I thought it might, I replied, but to my knowledge no one had ever been able to prove it. That's why, I said, it might be of importance to look at the wealth of information already collected.

Mr. Choate was still not satisfied. Didn't I know in which counties most infants were dying?

I told him that were more than 3,000 counties. Each county, moreover, listed death rates for white and "nonwhite" infants. It would take many more hours than I could spare to even rank every county in proper order. Even then, I pointed out, further investigation would be needed to see if, in those counties with the highest rates, a major amount of malnutrition existed.

Mr. Choate became exasperated. He'd asked a simple question, he said. But he'd received no answer at all. The government, he inferred, knew more than we were divulging. We had more facts than we would admit.

I told him that I wished such were indeed the case.

"Just send me the statistics," he said. "I'll analyze them."

I told him that the statistics were marked "Administrative Confidential" and I would have to check to see if they could be sent outside the department.

He was furious. He accused me of being uncooperative. He accused HEW of collecting data without any intention of using it. He accused the department of denying him information that should be available to any citizen upon request.

A disturbing thought crossed my mind. Robert Choate, I suddenly thought, viewed me in much the same light that I had viewed the Indian health director. He viewed me as a recalcitrant, inflexible bureaucrat—someone who refuses to divulge whatever information he possesses of a serious problem. Mr. Choate, I knew, wanted to publish a report on hunger in America. I seriously doubted that he employed any statisticians who could analyze the information sitting on my desk. I had little guarantee that HEW's computerized data—which, of course, were only numbers—would be used "responsibly." His report would cause even more furor than existed already. There would be more testimony and hearings. If he used the data to "prove" things that were unjustified, the department might be called to task.

On the other hand I knew he was right: HEW's statisticians had no intention of doing anything with the data. The computer print-outs had been sitting on a chair in my office gathering dust for several months now. I had never been able to interest anyone in studying them to see what, if anything, might be learned.

All these thoughts, and others, went through my mind.

"I'll send you the information," I said, finally. "Just remember," I added, "if you misuse it, it'll be your problem."

Robert Choate's report was published. There were more hearings. Federal officials held high-level meetings. But no one seemed to know how to proceed. Would a guaranteed income for food be best? A revamped food distribution program? Special food supplements for special people, such as pregnant women? Soybean protein packets for the poor? None of the officials seemed to have any idea which would be worth pursuing.

In the meantime it was taking HEW more than six months to begin its national nutrition survey—the exact same sort of survey that had already been done in more than thirty foreign countries. In fact, when Senator Joseph Clark wrote to HEW three months after Congress had ordered the survey to ask why funds had not yet been made available, it took the department two months to even answer his letter!

Two years later, HEW's survey had still only gathered "preliminary" results. At that time, moreover, it came to light that what was supposed to be a "national" survey included less than a dozen states. Congress was, to say the least, unpleasantly surprised.

"When the Congress authorized the National Nutrition Survey," a congressional committee complained, "it expected that survey to be completed within six months. Nearly two years have elapsed and it will be another six or more months before the complete results of the limited present ten-state survey are known."

Even HEW's limited survey, however, produced some disturbing "preliminary" results.

"The findings are as serious," testified Dr. Schaefer, "in the United States, if not more serious, than in many of the [foreign] countries we have studied."

How could such a disastrously serious situation have gone unnoticed for years in a country that boasts its conquest over fear from hunger? How could the inadequate nutrition of millions in America have gone unseen?

"This thing just fell between the cracks," said one experienced bureaucrat, when the dimensions of the malnutrition problem were becoming apparent.

"I am curious to know," Senator Percy asked Dr. Schaefer concerning HEW's nutrition survey, "why such a vital inquiry has not been initiated previously?" Why, the senator was asking, had the malnutrition problem fallen between the cracks?

"I don't know who one could blame," Schaefer replied, pondering the question for a moment, "except all the scientific community, the health authorities, I suppose Congress and all people . . . in making an assumption that we are in a land of plenty . . . we assume that in this sort of situation we will not find malnutrition."

Unfortunately Dr. Schaefer's mass indictment missed one important point. The malnutrition problem was not so much overlooked as it was "satisficed." The Agriculture Department thought it was doing a good enough job by merely doling out surplus food or food stamps, while ignoring the effect of these efforts on the nutrition of people. Federal officials thought they were doing a good enough job of assessing people's nutritional state by simply asking them about it. HEW was satisfied to study the problem where it was easiest to study, namely, in foreign countries rather than at home. Private industry took it for granted that by establishing its Nutrition Foundation it was doing enough about the problem. And finally, HEW's officials thought that a watered-down nutrition survey that took more than two years to yield "preliminary" facts would be adequate to assuage Congress.

The Department of Agriculture, in keeping with its lethargic interest in seeing whether or not Americans were being adequately fed, at first refused point-blank to put up any money for the HEW nutrition survey. Perhaps they thought it might uncover some things their own surveys had failed to find. During a meeting at the old Executive Office Building, where prehistoric fossils can be found in the floor tiles, an official of the Agriculture Department was asked if his department could put up an amount of money similar to that put up by HEW to start the survey.

"I think," he replied, "that my boss will refuse."

His boss was one of Secretary Freeman's assistants.

The agriculture officials knew that there was no real reason why they *had* to help support the nutrition survey. None of the congressmen on their appropriations committees—the committees that dole out money to agriculture programs—were even convinced that a problem existed and many were sure it didn't. "Why," the officials doubtlessly thought, "should we help finance a survey that might 'make waves' when our friends in Congress will be satisfied if we just keep doing what we've always done?"

Indeed this is exactly what happened. The agriculture officials, instead of trying to ferret out the answer to the question of how many Americans were malnourished, simply continued to publish more of the same reports that said the sort of things that have been said for years. Comfortable, easy-to-live-with reports that say, contrary to what we might expect, there is no difference between the diets of white and black children in Mississippi. At least, surveyed in the usual manner, there is no *detectable* difference.

The Agriculture Department's nutritionists—plump, middle-aged ladies in flower-print dresses—continue to flit about Washington in their spare time talking to women's clubs about leafy green vegetables or yellow tubers. Next year's report may be about to go to press. It will, no doubt, optimistically show that the diet of the "average American family" continues to improve. The flower-print ladies will have another chance to write a fine lengthy introduction in which the value of family nutrition education is stressed and the size of the monthly welfare food allowance is ignored. They will have a chance to talk about the nutritional value of green or pale-yellow vegetables. They may offer some well-meaning words on how the average "homemaker" can learn to help herself.

But while our officials continue to compose their annual "satisficing" reports, fewer Americans will be listening very closely. And some—the victims of America's unnoticed epidemic of hunger—may not be listening much longer at all.

# CHAPTER
## 7

*Four Million Dollars a Minute:*
*The Process Called Planning*

I had not been in Washington more than a few weeks, when I first heard someone say that the least desirable way for the government to operate is by reacting rapidly to pressing problems. Over and over, officials repeated the same lament—that they were too often forced to come up with quick answers to social problems. Too often, they complained, they had to respond in a limited amount of time to someone's inquiry.

"We do too much fire fighting around here," one administrator complained to me. "The White House wants a report on birth control by close of business today. Or the Bureau of the Budget wants to know how much we're spending on Indians by close of business tomorrow. Or some congressman wants to know how many one-eyed children there are in his district by close of business Friday. Most of our time is spent on this sort of stuff. Fire fighting. That's not what we should be here for."

Every official dreams not of day-to-day "fire fighting" but of planning, in a cool, orderly fashion for future problems. He dreams of anticipating and avoiding problems by careful planning. What's more, most people outside the government believe that such careful planning is continuously taking place. They believe that "extensive studies" of social problems are being carried out. They believe that, somewhere, someone is on top of the situation—that someone is trying to make sure that the benefits of our society are evenly spread around, trying to make sure that there is enough "room at the inn" for everyone.

During the time I spent in Washington I heard the virtues of planning extolled by numerous federal officials. Planning, in fact, seemed to be a hallowed word. Officials often went to great lengths to justify their faith in planning to skeptical citizens and congressmen.

"The concept of planning," said Surgeon General William Stewart in a speech, "has never been popular with Americans —largely, I think, because it has carried for many people the connotations of government, on the one hand, and of coercion on the other. As I have tried to make abundantly clear," General Stewart went on, "the kind of planning we envision provides coherent information on which to base democratic decision."

"Continuous and comprehensive planning is essential to the wise and economical development of health programs," said the deputy surgeon general at a congressional hearing.

One spring morning in 1967 a meeting took place at a plush motel in the Washington suburb of Bethesda. The agenda for this meeting has probably long since disappeared. The meeting itself was held in secret. No minutes or record of the proceedings were ever made public. There was not even a record kept of those who were participants.

Was the subject of this top secret gathering a new military defense system? A different policy for Southeast Asia? A new development in the space race?

The meeting was called to decide upon a national health plan.

In an atmosphere of secrecy that would put the CIA to shame, a national five-year health plan was to be decided upon.

Here is the story of this particular planning endeavor.

More than a year prior to this secret meeting President Johnson had ordered that plans for the next several years be prepared—not only for health, but also for all major domestic activities of the government. In response to this order, the surgeon general of the Public Health Service had set up a new office, to be run by his planning director, that was to prepare for his consideration the nation's first five-year health plan. The surgeon general ordered that the plan be finished in one year's time. When completed, the plan—it was expected—would show just how the Public Health Service might best deploy its efforts and its money over the next half decade in improving the nation's health.

A year later the surgeon general called a meeting of his budget committee to approve and "finalize" the new national health plan. The budget committee members, although no official list was ever available to the public, comprised the "top management" of the Public Health Service—the surgeon general and his immediate staff. The committee had always met in secret sessions. This year, however, secrecy was tighter than usual, perhaps because something new was expected from the meeting—a national five-year plan for bettering health. This year, in other words, the budget committee had to decide how to spend the funds given them by Congress for the next five years. They had to decide, for instance, how much of a yearly budget of some three-plus billion dollars would be spent on disease prevention, on training more health workers, on health research, and so forth. The eyes of many federal officials were focused on their Bethesda meeting to see what would emerge from a year's worth of intensive planning.

The meeting took place at the luxurious Linden Hill Hotel, a combination hotel-apartment overlooking the rolling Maryland countryside. Unlike previous budget committee meetings, it was not held on federal property, although numerous conference rooms were available in federal buildings throughout the Washington area. No observers were allowed. And as I said before, no transcript of the meeting was kept that has ever been made public.

The only way in which anyone can surmise what actually transpired at this secret all-day meeting is by carefully reading the document that emerged from it—the health plan. Today this document most likely cannot be located by even experienced and knowledgeable officials. It has long since probably disappeared in the quicksand of the bureaucracy. But it was a remarkable document indeed. It was, in many ways, a document that deserves careful study by anyone interested in the process called government planning.

The planners of Bethesda produced a document that rocked the federal establishment to its very foundations. Usually changes in spending for government programs are made by small degrees. A particular program will increase or decrease its budget by small amounts each year. These small increases or decreases are the end result of many pressures—political, economic, and other. The Bethesda health plan, however, was different. The plan proposed, among other things, that the federal government cut its spending for health research by 30 percent. The budget committee, after a year of "planning," produced a document that proposed to postpone such research projects as the artificial heart or a vaccine for cancer. It proposed to postpone research on the causes of mental retardation, strokes, and numerous other diseases. The plan proposed, in effect, to mark time in our research efforts and to spend the money in other ways.

No mention was made in the document of what kinds of research were to be curtailed or whether some sorts of research were to be given priority over other kinds. In fact no explanation of the committee's decision was given at all. The document did not state, for instance, that the nation is now supporting all those men who are capable of doing high-caliber research and that further spending for research would be a waste of money. It did not state that all the most important research problems were already under investigation, or that optimal progress was now being made.

This new plan for the next five years contained a number of other "decisions," none of which had any better justification than the one concerning research. No reasons for any of them were included. There was no mention in the document of how any of these decisions would affect the nation's health —supposedly the purpose of the plan. In fact there was nothing in the document to indicate that these choices on how to spend the taxpayers' dollars were not made by the toss of a coin or in some other equally arbitrary method.

What had gone awry with the planning process? A member of the surgeon general's planning staff explained to me what had happened.

"No national five-year plan exists," she said, when I expressed skepticism over the underlying basis for the budget committee's decisions. "Our office has never made any effort to produce one."

The staff member, an energetic young girl, waved her hand at a huge pile of paper on an adjoining desk. The pile contained several hundred copies of a speech recently given by the surgeon general's planning director.

"I spend all my time writing things like this," she said, handing me a copy. "They told me when I was hired that I was to work on policy planning—that's what my job description says—but I'm nothing but a speech writer with a fancy title."

I glanced at the first page of the director's speech.

"Planning in health," said one paragraph, "and in the Public Health Service, has come a long way in a very short time. . . ." I read further, "it is the planning *process* that is of paramount importance . . . a broad-based, orderly, organized, systematic process. . . ."

After a year of supposed planning—not to mention an expense of about one million dollars and the labor of some 50 trained staff members—the planning director had produced nothing that could be called a "plan." Despite the fact that a plan was urgently needed for the new federal budget, no one had ever gotten around to the arduous task of producing it. The surgeon general's planning director had spent a good part of his time traveling around the country making speeches about the necessity for planning. His highly trained staff had spent much of their time writing and editing these hortatory and erudite speeches. And in the meantime the national plan had remained unfinished.

"There is no five-year plan," the young girl staff member repeated. "The decisions that came out of that meeting have no basis at all." The decision to cut back on spending for health research, she explained, was a perfect example. None of the "planners" on the budget committee had any knowledge whatsoever of the nation's future research needs. They had never sought or received any advice about the problem. It may well have been true that too much money was being spent for research. Bu the planners had no way of knowing this. These men—though perhaps well intentioned—were totally ignorant of the facts they needed to know to complete their five-year plan.

The planners had never even bothered to find out, for instance, how much research of various types had already been planned. The National Institutes of Health—the federal multimillion dollar research agency—had already made a five-year plan. This plan had been printed in a document several inches thick. It had been sent to the surgeon general. In it the researchers outlined in great detail just what they hoped to accomplish over the next five years and what they thought their plans would cost.

In fact at the very moment the budget committee met at the Linden Hill Hotel, this research plan reposed in the office of the surgeon general's planning director. Unfortunately neither he nor anyone concerned with formulating the five-year health plan had ever gotten around to reading it. No person at the budget committee's secret meeting had ever read it. Like most government documents, it had never been used despite the thousands of man-hours consumed in its making.

The only difference was in this instance the NIH plan had *supposedly* been taken into account in preparing the overall national plan. The surgeon general's planners had supposedly used it to construct their five-year plan. Nonetheless these men—with sublime confidence—went ahead to recommend a 30 percent decrease in research spending. They went ahead —without having made any preparation for their decision— to vote to postpone the development of an artificial heart or a cancer vaccine, both of which were specifically mentioned in the NIH plan.

I glanced at the planning director's fine-sounding speech again.

"Planning in health, and in the Public Health Service, has come a long way in a very short time . . . it is the planning *process* that is of paramount importance . . . a broad-based, organized, systematic process. . . ."

I could easily see why most people were skeptical about the process our officials call "planning." I could see why people might be skeptical of the sort of "broad-based, orderly systematic" planning process that was utilized to arrive at the decisions made in Bethesda that morning, skeptical of what role Surgeon General Stewart's "democratic decision" played at that secret Bethesda planning meeting, of which no records were ever kept, skeptical of what use the surgeon general's planners made of the "coherent information" reposing in his own office, but ignored in the making of his national health plan.

There is nothing so disappointing as a public official who says the right things in his speeches but seems incapable of bringing his actions up to the high standards he has preached. Perhaps General Stewart and his planners should have tried their hands at the sort of planning they spoke about, before making all their fine-sounding speeches.

It's no wonder that the word "planning" raises the hackles of many a congressman. It is no wonder that the term has long been in disrepute and will continue to be as long as planning is done the way it was done in Bethesda that morning. The men who sat in the Bethesda hotel that spring morning are the sort of men who give the process called planning a bad name. Yet in most cases these are the same men who pay such lip service to the need for planning. The men who met to decide on a national health plan were not planners. They had no knowledge of real planning—planning that springs from the needs of people and is geared to meet those needs. They were and are, since many are still in high government positions, men who like to meddle with the lives and futures of others without even taking the responsibility —not to mention the time to prepare—for doing so.

To this day no roster of the men who participated in that planning meeting can be found. The decisions they made were made in total anonymity. There is no record of who favored or disfavored the decisions, or why. The document containing them was circulated throughout the government as the end product of a year's worth of planning that had never, in fact, been carried out.

Ironically I found as I talked to more government workers involved in planning that the surgeon general's planning director was in actuality correct. Federal planning *had* come a long way in a very short time. Actually the shoddy Bethesda effort at planning *was* an improvement over the manner in which most federal programs up to that time had operated. Up until only recently, in fact, there had hardly been even a pretense toward planning in our social programs. So haphazardly were these programs planned that their advisory councils invariably met in secret sessions—just as the budget committee did that morning—and kept no detailed records. Anyone outside the government was hard put to fathom the basis for their "decisions."

Even "insiders"—I came to realize—were frequently unclear about how the programs they were supposed to be running should be planned. In 1967, for instance, a new program was launched. It was to provide for a nationwide network of urban centers to improve the welfare of mothers and children. But as so often happens, the program's "planners" were faced with a dilemma: which cities were to get a center? With limited funds and many applicants expected, some basis for selecting the cities were needed. A long list of "criteria" was drawn up. It included such considerations as how well the city in question had worked with federal agencies in the past or whether the city possessed a major university. Oddly enough—in the entire list—no mention was given to how serious the social problems were in the city that the urban center was designed to combat.

"What do you intend to emphasize most," I asked one of the officials responsible for planning this program, "in deciding which cities are to get funds for a center?"

"We intend," he replied, "to place greatest emphasis on local capability to mount the rapid effort needed to get the centers under way." What he meant, in other words, was that those cities that already had the most abundant local resources—including already existing federal programs—would most likely be those cities rewarded with still another federal project.

In most federal programs this sort of upside-down logic is what passes for planning. Most programs give their money to reputable and established institutions or individuals that, it is felt, will do a good job. Whether or not the people who live in the locales in which these institutions or men are working happen to need the project more than people who live elsewhere is something else again.

The results of this brand of upside-down planning are exactly what one might expect. Philadelphia at last count had some half-dozen projects trying to do the exact same thing for the welfare of mothers and children *funded by the same federal agency.* New Orleans, without demonstrably less need, had none.

The absence of planning based on people's needs is the rule, not the exception, in our social programs. And this explains why we aren't getting our effort's worth—not to mention our money's worth—from these programs. Our planners have yet to appreciate, evidently, that local areas with the greatest needs should probably receive the greatest efforts. Areas with the worst health levels, for instance, should get priority for health efforts and areas with the worst educational levels deserve priority in our education programs. There are obviously other things to be taken into account, but at present not even the most meager attempt is made to plan on the basis of local needs such as these.

Right now it looks as though no planning is going on at all. A study of the government's program to train teachers concluded that those localities where education was worst benefited least from the government's effort to train better teachers. A recent study of high school dropouts and adult illiteracy in 131 American cities concluded that no relation at all could be found between the amount or character of education or welfare programs and the amount of school failure and illiteracy in each city. A study of the government's hospital building program could find no relation between where hospitals are being built and health levels. The Citizen's Board of Inquiry found that those local areas where hunger and starvation were probably worst benefited least from government food programs.

The lack of planning shows also in the nearly total absence of any coordination between programs. Hospitals are built without any plans for staffing them. Housing developments are built in places where no jobs or social services are available. Men are trained for jobs that don't exist or encouraged to seek jobs where housing doesn't exist.

The very structure of the government with its thousands of independent bureaus and offices makes this mess inevitable —especially if nothing is done to correct it. Most program managers wouldn't know whom they should coordinate with, even if they wanted to. Instead, in quiet desperation, they fall back on doing "their own thing" as best they can.

Since no planning is being done, it would probably make as much sense to dole out federal funds for social programs on the basis of the number of people in each state or local area as in any other manner. Indeed this is exactly what happens in hundreds of programs. Congress, unwilling to trust the bureaucrats to plan, has devised hundreds of different formulas to dole out funds to states and localities. Most of these formulas are based on such rudimentary criteria as the number of people who live in the area and their income. The formulas have, in most cases, no relation to people's needs; many, in fact, have not been changed for twenty years or more. Thanks to these formulas, it can truthfully be said that —for better or worse—most of the government's domestic programs "run themselves." For better or worse most social programs are run by rote, unencumbered by any human planning whatsoever. Most of our social programs could be quite successfully managed by any mathematically inclined high school student.

There are, in fact, so many formulas for doling out federal funds that even top officials themselves don't know how many exist.

"Oh, I would say a hundred and fifty," replied HEW's Secretary Cohen, when asked how many of these algebraic rules his department used. "And I think that is probably on the low side," he said.

One large area where planning has been least apparent is the area of spending for research. The Department of Health, Education and Welfare, for example, spent more than a billion dollars last year on research. Unfortunately the vast majority of these research projects were undertaken without any thought on the part of federal officials as to whether they were really needed or of what use their results might be. They were, in effect, "research for research's sake" with no planning whatsoever.

The study of poverty is a good example. As soon as it became fashionable, and even lucrative, to study poverty, corps of researchers cropped up in every university and "think tank" across the country. Reams of studies were generated with generous federal support. Many of these studies were voluminous and made difficult bedtime reading. In addition, most of them were worthless. Students of poverty produced huge tomes that sought to relate poverty to other things. We can learn from poring over these tomes, for instance, that poor people in almost any city in America have less schooling than other people. That they have poorer health and poorer nutrition. That they are more likely to have had poor parents and grandparents. That they are more likely to live in poor housing.

Our government, and many private agencies, paid millions of dollars each year for studies such as these. Some of them were quite sophisticated. They made use of computers and contained lots of complex equations. But when all is said and done, all of these sorts of studies left their readers with the same question—the question of cause and effect. Which came first—poverty or poor education, poor housing, poor health, and so forth? How much of a change in one will be followed by a change in the others?

These chicken-and-egg studies were worthless in trying to answer such questions. A study of hospital care, for instance, showed that poor people used more hospital care than other people. The authors thought their research had uncovered something "surprising." But what did this "discovery" actually mean? Did it mean that the poor used more hospital care because they were sicker? Or that the hospitals the poor used were worse than others and thus that their patients stayed longer? Did it mean that, to improve their health, poor people needed more, or less, hospital care?

Such a study tells us nothing about how to ameliorate human problems. It merely presents us with an "interesting" or "surprising" situation. It is research for the sake of research. We have many such studies. We have lots of studies that tell us that poor people are more likely to have had poor grandparents, but few studies that tell us how we can prevent their having poor children. We have too few tryouts and experiments in social progress. We have practically no studies that seek to show how many infant lives can be saved by better health care. Or how many convicts can be kept from returning to prison through better rehabilitation programs. We have far too few trial projects that show just how much we can eliminate poor reading by reducing classroom size or by better teaching. Or how much mental illness we can prevent by less crowded housing.

For many years, for example, we've known that overcrowded housing is highly associated with certain human problems. "Poor housing," wrote Alvin Schorr, a former HEW official, "correlates to a high degree with rates of illness and death, with the rate of mental illness, with juvenile and adult delinquency, and with many other social problems. . . ." Yet despite our great concern with these problems—not to mention their great waste in terms of human life and potential— none of our federal housing programs have ever tried to see whether juvenile delinquency, for example, could be diminished by providing better, less crowded housing. Or by different styles of housing. Or by anything else. As a result, we haven't the slightest idea whether we can decrease delinquency by providing a different type of living environment. We have just gone along doing what we have always done, while the problem gets no better. We have wasted precious time and have wasted human lives as well.

If the proper study of mankind is man, our federal research dollars have obviously been buying studies of something else. They have been buying studies of phenomena such as "poverty" or "social status" or "illiteracy" or the relation between them. But they have not been buying studies that indicate how to change human problems for the better. They have not been buying studies of how far-flung programs affect human beings and their problems.

How, for instance, do federal programs affect American families? Despite the well-meaning words of politicians and officials on the desirability of promoting family life, the government has never really tried to see how well its social programs affect family stability or family life in general. Almost no government programs deal with entire families at all, but with individuals instead. Some, it almost seems, were even designed to purposefully disrupt family life and make it harder for people to stay together.

A few years ago it was found that widows receiving Social Security benefits lost their benefits if they remarried. This odd quirk of law had led to many widows living "in sin" with prospective husbands rather than risk loss of their Social Security benefits. Yet this situation was uncovered, not by federal officials, but by congressmen receiving irate letters from their constituents.

The AFDC program—the welfare program for poor mothers and their children—is another example. This program has frequently been said to encourage the breakup of families. Yet, as Mr. Schorr pointed out, few officials or for that matter social scientists have seemed interested in finding out whether or not this assertion is true. Schorr put it this way:

> Was it said that AFDC tends to break up families? In 1959, researchers had not explored the matter and did not seem to know. Indeed, the relevant portion of the law had been amended, offering an unequaled opportunity for research, *but no one troubled.* (Emphasis added.)

Does AFDC tend to break up families? Today, as in 1959, virtually none of our officials or social researchers have troubled to find out. The same is true of all our other programs—their impact on family life remains a mystery, although we have many hints that certain programs may operate to destroy, rather than enhance, family life.

What happens to the results of whatever government-supported research *is* carried out to completion?

"I don't know of any use ever made of my research," a well-known economist told me. "I've never even heard if anyone read my report."

I once asked Dr. Harald Graning, the head of the government's hospital construction agency, which spends some three hundred million dollars a year, if he knew of a certain project his agency had sponsored. This highly elaborate project had been going on for several years. It dealt with the problem of estimating the costs of the various services for which his agency was trying to provide facilities. The project's results were about to be published by a major university and it was undoubtedly the most important research project his agency was funding. Yet the agency head had no knowledge of the project whatsoever. He was totally unaware that research was going on in this area, let alone research funded by his own agency.

Examples of this sort of sublime ignorance of the results of government-supported research are legion. One day I received a call from a friend, a woman researcher at Washington's Children's Hospital. She told me a strange story. HEW, she said, had been supporting her research project, to the tune of about $100,000, for the past several years. Now she had heard that the government was about to cut off its support, despite the fact that her research had already resulted in a promising cure for the most common known cause of mental retardation. Her research results had been published in a leading journal and presented at professional meetings. Yet she had never been asked to present the results of her research to federal officials, though she had offered to do so. And she was unable to find out why her funds were being cut off.

Almost in desperation, she had called me to see if I could do anything to help.

I telephoned the director of HEW's mental retardation program. He knew nothing about the project.

"It must be," I said, "one of the most expensive projects your program is supporting." He agreed, but still denied any knowledge of it.

I asked him if he were aware of the project's initially favorable results or of the potential significance of these results.

I asked him how many mentally retarded individuals might be affected if the project proved successful. He had no idea. He was not even aware of how much money had been invested in the project to date or how much might be needed to carry it to completion.

It is considered highly improper in HEW for anyone to try to influence any decision concerning a scientific, or research grant. The director was, of course, quite aware of *this* fact.

"What interest do you have in this project," he asked me, belligerently.

His tone made it quite clear that he regarded my interest as interference, even though I had asked only about the merits of the project and had deliberately avoided asking whether or not it would be re-funded. The mental retardation director's ignorance, as well as his suggestion that I was meddling where I had no right to, so annoyed me that I telephoned several friends in the department with an interest in mental retardation.

"Make some waves," I told them. "Try to find out what's going on."

My aim was to let the director know that—whatever decision he made—enough interest existed inside the department that it might have to be justified to someone besides himself and his staff. His decision could not simply be one made in secret or by default. This strategy must have worked for I eventually heard that the project's funds had been continued for another year.

In addition, I earned the lasting enmity of the mental retardation director, an official who was totally unaware of the results of research supported by his agency that promised to cure the leading known cause of mental retardation and who, moreover, was unaware that the project had been refused further support by his agency for the coming year and was in danger of being scrapped for lack of money.

Imagine the secretary of the Air Force being unaware of the development of a new fighter plane. Or the secretary of the Navy of a new type of nuclear submarine. Yet this is precisely what is going on right now in our social programs. Our administrators are unaware of the results of research, funded by their own agencies, directed to the very same problems they are supposedly trying to solve.

One reason why our administrators are in the dark is because there is no easy way for them to find out what research their agency, or any other, has done. No file of research results exists. There is not even any record of whether or not a particular project was completed successfully or not.

A researcher recently sent in a six-month progress report. In his report he informed Washington that the same research he was carrying out was being done by two other researchers under grants from the same agency!

His honesty is commendable. If he had not brought this fact to the attention of government officials, they would never have found out. In fact, if instead he had simply inquired about what research was being done in his field, it would have taken Washington several weeks to come up with an answer, and even then it would most likely have been an incomplete one.

A great portion of our government's non-defense research concerns health and environmental problems. The National Institutes of Health, for instance, spend about a billion dollars each year. All of this research is done with hardly even any pretense toward planning. In fact, until a few years ago, the NIH director did not even have a planning staff. The officials running our health research program seemed content to let the program run itself. Several years ago Congress was sold on the idea that a blank check for our nation's scientists would be the best way to improve our nation's health and life in general. Congress was led down the primrose path by scientists who said, in effect, "Just give us lots of money, leave us alone, and we'll produce lots of research breakthroughs."

Unfortunately this strategy was a failure. Certain vital areas of research were completely neglected despite the clear need for attention. Problems such as emphysema and automobile accidents were almost totally ignored by researchers until congressmen started wondering if anything could be done to stem the thousands of yearly deaths they caused. Officials doled out millions of dollars to discover what goes on inside a red blood cell, but virtually nothing to find out why one-third of all blood collected each year spoils on the shelf. They spent millions to develop an artificial kidney, but practically nothing to try to make it inexpensive enough so that more than a fraction of those who need it could afford it.

How could our officials pour billions into finding out what goes on inside cells and spend virtually nothing to discover better ways to supply even rudimentary services to people? One reason is simply that, because our research programs have never been planned, no person in the government has even known how much research is being done on cells as opposed to people. Or animals versus people. If the figures were known, they would probably surprise even the government planners.

If any research "breakthroughs" have occurred, it is certainly not the doing of those officials who have administered the spending of public funds for health research. A study of the multimillion-dollar health research program came to this conclusion about how much planning was being done by the officials responsible for this program:

> "Planning" is perhaps the rubric under which the Panel should mention its perplexity over the apparent absence of any obvious ... intense concern to apply the results of biomedical research to improve human health and longevity. ... The Panel wonders how any competing claims of applied research arise, who hears the debate, and how the decisions are reached.

One November afternoon I got a lesson in just how unplanned a federal research program could be. I attended a meeting of an advisory council whose members were supposed to advise federal officials on what was called the General Research Support (GRS) Program. Under this unique program research institutions received federal dollars simply because they were already doing a certain amount of government-sponsored research. The whole process worked—and still works—exactly like a television quiz show bonus jackpot and with just as much forethought and planning on the part of the officials running the program.

A congressional subcommittee, disturbed at the nebulous purposes of this program, had issued a report containing this opinion:

> The committee is surprised by the casualness with which the GRS program has been administered . . . it is disquieting . . . to find policies so vague. . . .

Less than a month after this report appeared, the advisory council met to help HEW officials award more GRS grants. At this meeting, however—possibly because of the congressional report—some council members put up a fuss. They complained that the program administrators were using them as "rubber stamps." They were not being given enough facts to make intelligent choices among the institutions that applied for money.

One member tried to get the GRS program's administrators to clarify the purpose of the "advice" he was supposed to give them:

> What I am asking is . . . the general purpose of the program . . . the specific issues you feel exist . . . providing a framework within which one could then assess the particular grant. . . .

The council member was asking, in effect, what yardsticks he was to use in deciding which research institutions were to get the program's funds. He was asking what the program was supposed to accomplish.

The council member quickly found, however, that the GRS administrators were not at home talking about the purposes of their program. They could, he found, wax eloquent about the "freedom of science" and the "unfettered purpose of sci-

entific investigation" but when it came to talking about the
purposes of their program they were strangely inarticulate.
Here is how the program's administrator replied to the council member who, by law, was supposed to advise him on how
to best spend the program's money:

> This thing (GRS) has become ritualistic now. Each
> year institutions . . . have to show they have been suc-
> cessful in winning 100,000 dollars of . . . support. . . .

Hardly an answer that elucidates the research program's
goals. After a few other such vague remarks the council member who had sought to discover what yardsticks he was to
use in "advising" the government on how to spend its funds
gave up in disgust. It seemed that the officials in charge of
running the program didn't know themselves—or wouldn't
divulge—what its purpose was. That afternoon the council
approved the awarding of grants to more than 250 institutions without any idea why these, and not 250 others, had
been selected.

"Very fine" said the council chairman, when this parody of
decision making was over.

"We spent . . ." he said, contentedly, "forty-one million dollars in about nine minutes."

I suddenly realized that the chairman who was boasting so
glibly of spending more than four million dollars a minute
was none other than the same person who had characterized
the government's planning process as "a broad-based, orderly,
organized, systematic" one. He was none other than the surgeon general's planning director. This official, after the council had spent forty-one million dollars, gave a little speech to
try, as he said, to "put things in perspective" for his advisers.
His words tell a good deal about why planning in the government is at a standstill:

> . . . the $41 million is very large, indeed, but in trying
> to develop a Council with the major authority and re-
> sponsibility the Department is asking you to worry
> about $3 billion annually and as the department re-

organization takes place, if it goes along the line that many hope, it will be a concern for $10 billion.

The planning director went on in his attempt to reassure the council that their "advice" would be needed even more in the future, if things were to go the way that "many" hoped:

> I am not certain I can really comprehend that amount of money, but I know it is a lot larger than $41 million, which I can't comprehend either.

The planning director was, of course, foremost among the many who were hoping, as the department was being reorganized, to gain the power for planning—with the "advice" of his council—for all health programs. And while his too humble words may have comforted some of the council members, one can only wonder how comforting they would be to the average American citizen and taxpayer. How comforting, for instance, would they be to thousands of hungry schoolchildren for whom forty-one million dollars could buy decent lunches each day? How comforting to thousands of mothers living in poverty for whom forty-one million dollars could help pay for job training or for day care for their children? And just to put matters in perspective a bit more, one can only wonder how comforting it would be to Americans to realize that, since its inception the GRS program had spent, not forty-one million dollars but several hundred million dollars in the same hasty, haphazard manner.

The planning director may have been pleased with his council and their day's work—but it is unlikely that anyone else would consider it worth the price of flying the members to and from Washington. How can any sensible person view such a spectacle with anything but the utmost contempt? How can anyone take this sort of government tomfoolery as anything but a farcical display? The conclusion anyone must reach about an advisory council that can dispense forty-one million dollars in nine minutes is that the process is more than "ritualistic." It is downright sleight of hand.

The whole business reminded me of a story told me by a

wealthy dollar-a-year official. "You know," he is supposed to
have said, "you lose all perspective working for the government. You get so that you think a hundred thousand dollars
mean nothing. But my father used to work a whole day to
make a hundred thousand."

Perhaps the joke is no laughing matter after all. Perhaps
our officials—like the planning director—*have* lost all sense of
the import of the millions of dollars they giddily dispense
each day. It's no wonder with this sort of person planning
our government's social programs that these programs are in
such a sorry state. Little wonder, with this sort of haphazard
planning going on in our agencies devoted to social progress,
that—no matter how noble their aims—their programs are
doomed to failure.

I remember wondering, as the government advisers filed
out of their meeting on the GRS program, whether a roomful
of our poorest citizens, perhaps those from the Poor People's
Campaign who had petitioned the government for greater
representation for the poor on government planning and advisory councils, would have spent forty-one million dollars in
nine minutes. Perhaps not being expert planners, it might
have taken them somewhat longer. Perhaps in their inexper-
tise they might have been less hasty in dispensing such a
sum. As I watched the GRS administrators hastily pack their
thick briefcases, relieved at having gotten through another
advisory council meeting, I wondered whether a group of
our poorest citizens would have allowed them to escape so
easily without explaining what they thought their program's
goals really were.

Better planning may indeed be the magic panacea for our
officials. But anyone who has seen what masquerades under
the name of "planning" in the secret meetings of budget committees from which meaningless documents emerge, anyone
who has sat and watched the government's advisers spend millions of dollars in a few moments, anyone who has witnessed
these fumbling efforts can hardly help wondering whether
perhaps more than just a little *better* planning is needed.

# CHAPTER
# 8

## *The Computation of Compassion*

Ask anyone which federal agency has done the most for social progress in the past few years. Most would name the
Department of Health, Education and Welfare or one of its
dozens of subagencies. Some might say the Office of Economic Opportunity, which runs the poverty program. A few
might nominate the Department of Labor, for its efforts to
provide training and jobs.

The answer is most likely none of these.

Our federal agency has probably done more than any
other for the cause of social progress during the past five
years. It has done what no other department or bureau has
been able to do. It has shown us how the solution of social
problems can be planned and carried out.

That agency is the Department of Defense.

There is nothing mysterious or secret about what the Defense Department has done about social problems here in
America. It has taught us how to tackle them. It has given

our nation's so-called social planners a much-needed lesson in problem solving.

One morning in November of 1967 then Secretary of Defense Robert McNamara gave one of his lesser-known speeches. It was not about our "assured destruction capability" or our antiballistic missile system. It was a speech not about what the Department of Defense had done to destroy life but on what it had done to enhance it. Mr. McNamara's words made few headlines, but they were remarkable words indeed.

"I want to talk to you this morning," he began, "about the unused potential of the Department of Defense—a potential for contributing to the solution of the social problems racking our nation." Can the vast resources of the Defense Department, the secretary asked his audience, "be used to contribute to our nation's benefit beyond the narrow, though vitally necessary, role of military power?" After posing this question, Mr. McNamara then went on to describe certain ways in which the Department of Defense—an institution whose primary responsibility is to maintain the military posture of the country—had become involved in helping what the secretary called "the social profile" of the nation and to tell his audience about three projects initiated by the Defense Department to combat social problems: a program to promote off-base open housing for military personnel; a program to train poverty youths for productive careers; and finally a program to aid servicemen in finding jobs after their discharge from the armed forces.

The Secretary of Defense's speech may not have amazed many of his listeners. But it did not fail to impress some of his fellow officials. Copies of the speech were widely circulated in Department of Health, Education and Welfare and elsewhere. The Defense Department's "social" programs caused quite a stir, especially among those familiar with the sluggish pace of most of our other social programs.

"What *this* Department needs," a young HEW official said to me, after reading a copy of the speech, "is a Robert Mc-

Namara. He's done more in a year," he said, "than most of our programs have done in the last decade."

Mr. McNamara told his audience that November morning, first, about the progress the Defense Department had made toward solving the problem of racial discrimination in off-base servicemen's housing. "In northern Virginia and Maryland," he said, "within 120 days we more than tripled the number of nondiscriminatory units—from 15,000 to 53,000 units."

Very few of his listeners probably appreciated the magnitude of this achievement. Few probably realized, for instance, that in four months Mr. McNamara opened about as many dwelling units to his servicemen as our entire federal urban renewal agency—which does not even have a *plan* for urban desegregation—*built* in its entire first decade. Very few of his audience probably knew that it took the Housing Assistance Administration, the agency responsible for more than half a million public housing units, nearly *one year* after the 1964 Civil Rights Act became law to draw up guidelines for desegregating these units.

Robert McNamara had still more to tell. He spoke about his department's attempts to train men—men whom society had passed by as hopeless—for jobs they could do in military and then in civilian life. He spoke about a new program to train men formerly rejected as unfit for military service—Project 100,000:

> The goal of Project 100,000 was . . . to take in 40,000 rejectees the first year, and 100,000 each year thereafter . . . we took 49,000 . . . more than half these men . . . in poverty.

Again, the magnitude of this simply stated feat probably escaped his audience. They may not have appreciated the fact that Project 100,000 tackled, in its first year, the training and rehabilitation of about half as many men as the poverty program's major ongoing effort, the Job Corps, did in 1968. And, as though that were not enough, Mr. McNamara described another program—Project Transition—that sought to help an additional 750,000 men who leave the armed forces each year to find civilian training and jobs.

It is likely that morning that no one in the audience—a gathering of educational television broadcasters—recognized the magnitude of the achievements that Mr. McNamara described. There was probably no one who appreciated the fact that in just over one year the Defense Department had done more to ameliorate the stubborn problem of housing discrimination than all other federal agencies combined, including the Department of Housing and Urban Development, *had ever done*. In about the same time it had shouldered the responsibility for training and assisting as many young men as were being trained in all our other manpower programs put together.

It is easy to brush these feats aside. It is easy to be cynical about them. But when we look at the fumbling attempts of many of our other agencies, both in and outside of government, to solve the same problems, one becomes less cynical. We must face the fact that, in not a few ways, our most destructive agency is doing as much or more for the causes of social progress than any other agency. We must face the fact that while our officials fumble and produce piles of guidelines and memoranda, our most "non-humane" agency seems rapidly able to pinpoint and address these problems.

Faced with this reality, one gets less cynical—and more inquisitive. Why is this so? What was Robert McNamara's secret method?

The reasons for Secretary McNamara's success in tackling social problems were less complex than many supposed. His method was straightforward and sensible. First, Mr. McNamara and his staff—unlike most of our other officials— tried to get some idea of the size of the problems they faced before they tackled them. Before they tried, for instance, to desegregate off-base housing they first made a nationwide survey of rental practices. They established the actual size of the problem. "We sent teams to a dozen bases to look into every aspect of equal opportunity. . . ." Mr. McNamara explained. "Seventeen thousand service families were surveyed. Their answers were analyzed."

Mr. McNamara and his staff also sized up the magnitude of the problem that Project 100,000 was designed to tackle—the problem of drafting and training men formerly considered untrainable. They concluded after this assessment that:

> though . . . 1.8 million young men [reach] military service age each year in the United States, some 600,000 —a full third—were failing to qualify under our draft standards. . . . In some areas, the failure rate . . . ran as high as 60 percent; and for Negroes in some states it exceeded 80 percent.

For Project Transition, designed to help men leaving the service find jobs, the Defense Department's chief assessed the size of the problem with similar diligence:

> We surveyed the situation, and found that some 50 percent of the men about to leave the services need and want some degree of help to make the transition to a productive civilian life.

Sizing up the problem may not seem like such a novel technique. It may seem merely sensible. But when we look at how little is known about the extent of most social problems, about where they are worst or becoming worse, Mr. McNamara's attempt to assess the size and location of these problems represents a radical departure from the sort of social planning that has been taking place in our other federal agencies. Our health planners have no idea where various health problems—adult mortality for example—are most serious or are getting worse. Our education officials share the same ignorance when it comes to reading levels or dropout rates. The men who run our job training programs have little idea where the most men who want and need training are. Officials in charge of juvenile delinquency don't know what cities have the most delinquents or where delinquency is becoming a worse problem.

When the massive multimillion-dollar Model Cities program began in 1967 it was supposed to make an effort— for the first time—at making broad social improvement in urban areas. It was supposed to make sure that government money spent in these areas would be spent where the problems were most serious. The government's officials were to make sure that each city's application for funds painted an accurate picture of just how serious the city's problems were —and how serious one city's problems were in comparison with those of another.

Dozens of applications came in from cities all over the nation. Stacked one on top of the other in their powder-blue covers, they would have reached from ceiling to floor. They were packed up and, along with some federal urban experts, were carted off to a suburban "retreat" where for several days the officials tried to decide which cities most deserved the money.

"It was hell," said one, "trying to decide how one city stacked up against another in terms of where the problems were worst. There was just no way to tell which areas were worse off in particular ways—education, health, employment opportunities, and so forth. In fact," he concluded, "the real problem is going to come when we try to decide, ten years from now, whether there's been any real improvement. Unless we get the base-line information that tells us where we are now, there won't be any way to even guess."

Viewed in this light it is easy to see why Mr. McNamara's approach to problem solving was so novel. Not only did he first try to estimate the size of the problems but he then set up ways to see if his programs were really helping to improve the situation.

After establishing the size of the problem, Mr. McNamara decided what he wanted his new programs to accomplish. He set goals and specific targets on the way to these goals. In his housing and manpower efforts he established criteria for success at each step of the way. In housing, for example, a goal was a certain number of housing units freed from discrimination, "nondiscriminatory units," as he called them. In training there were still other goals—the number of servicemen placed in civilian jobs, and so forth. If Robert McNamara had a secret weapon in his battle against the same social problems that have so effectively stymied our other officials, it was in part his ability to chart his progress in an objective way. The secret weapon was a careful evaluation of what was really being accomplished.

His constant evaluation of the progress of his social efforts paid off. Project 100,000 surpassed its goal of 40,000 rejectees trained in its first year by 9,000 men. It met other important goals as well. "The successful graduation rate [from basic training] of these 49,000 was 96 percent," said the secretary.

"We are launching," he went on, "a careful follow-up study to test conclusively the ultimate outcome of Project 100,000. At least a decade of careful measurement of the performance of the men both in and out of the service will be required."

Robert McNamara's ten-year follow-up of "graduates" from the Defense Department's training program was the first such effort in government—the first time any administrator had gone to such great lengths to really see if what he is doing really means better lives for the people affected.

Trying to judge the success of most government programs is, as someone once said, like trying to make love to an octopus. It almost seems as though these programs have been purposefully designed to resist evaluation. Many, like the multibillion-dollar welfare program, let the several states operate in such an infinity of ways—often without even informing the federal government—that the sheer chaos of the program makes it impossible to evaluate its success. The Medicaid program, welfare's health care program, is so different in every state that it is impossible for anyone to say which are doing the best jobs.

Nearly every federal program—to make matters worse—collects reams of statistics—but invariably the key facts that would allow someone to judge whether or not the program is accomplishing its goals are missing. The Housing Act of 1949 is a good example. This twenty-year-old law establishing the federal urban renewal program set forth several original goals. Among other things the program was supposed to be set up:

> to eliminate substandard and other inadequate housing through clearance of slums and other blighted areas . . .

> to stimulate housing production and community development sufficient to remedy the housing shortage . . .

> to realize the goal of a decent home and a suitable living environment for every American family. . . .

These noble goals have been repeated and restated many times since 1949. No one would quarrel with their basic intent. But can we tell if the urban renewal program—or any other program, for that matter—is attaining these goals?

Do we know enough about the twenty-year-old urban renewal program to judge whether or not it is attaining any of its goals? The answer is discouraging. Martin Anderson, a long-time student of urban renewal, tells us that, incredible as it may seem, "There are no published figures available concerning the number of new dwelling units that were built with urban renewal areas. . . ."

To make matters worse, Anderson says:

> We don't even know the exact number of people involved in the federal urban renewal program . . . the Urban Renewal Administration published data on only the number of families. . . . Thus we cannot be sure whether the families we are talking about consist of two people or ten people.

There is virtually no information, on a nationwide scale, about what happens to people and families displaced by urban renewal. We have no idea—at least from the facts the federal program gathers—about whether these people are living in better or worse circumstances than before they were displaced. We do know from a variety of limited local studies that in most cases the "living environment" of these displaced families is worse after urban renewal than before—they pay higher rents, live in more dilapidated housing, and have higher rates of illness and dependency. But no data collected by federal officials would give us any idea whether the "living environment" of urban renewal families is being bettered by the program. In fact we know little about the "living environment" of American families in general. Our most recent nationwide estimate of the number of substandard homes was made ten years ago. We have never even tried to estimate for the nation the amount of overcrowding that exists. We know virtually nothing about any of the other things that most of us would agree militate against a suitable living environment. How many families live in homes infested by rats, roaches, and other vermin or live with too much noise? We haven't the faintest idea on a nationwide scale of the answers to these simple questions.

How well is the urban renewal program accomplishing the ambitious goals it set in 1949? The conclusion is that *there is no way to tell.* We can only guess. Our guess can hardly be an optimistic one. We can hardly be sanguine about how well the program is bettering the living environment of the American family. But the simple fact is our officials have made no attempt to evaluate the program in terms of the goals it set for itself twenty years ago.

Our other programs are no better. Our hospital building program is twenty years old too. It began with the high-minded goal of "assuring an adequate amount of services" to all people who couldn't afford to pay for them. Now—two decades later—the program's managers have no idea how successful they have been in attaining this goal. The several-year-old school lunch program has no idea how successful if has been in serving lunches to poor children. In fact it doesn't even know how many poor children it serves now. The government's mental retardation program is another example. Begun by President Kennedy, it was to show that the mentally retarded can lead useful and productive lives. Today—five years after its start—its managers barely know how many people the program serves, let alone what is being done for them. What is more, they have no serious plans for gathering any of this information. They are seemingly content to just sit back and let the program "run itself."

The list of programs that have set ambitious goals, and have no idea how well they are attaining them, could go on and on. Many of these programs are several decades old. But regardless of their age virtually none of our social programs has made vigorous ongoing attempts at self-evaluation.

The reason for this lack of long-term information on how well our social programs are working is simply that the men who manage these programs have never tried to see how well they are accomplishing their goals—if they have any idea what those goals are. Many officials, in fact, have never even thought very much about the purposes of their programs. An administrator whose program was one designed to provide money for the construction of research facilities, for example, could think of no other measure of the program's success than the "millions of square feet" of space that had been built. Ask an administrator how well his program is working and he will most likely tell you how many grants were awarded, how many institutions received funds, or the total number of "centers" for such-and-such a purpose that were built. Beyond these simpleminded ways of judging a program's success, the average administrator does not seem to be able to go.

The fact that most of these programs spend several millions of dollars each year doesn't seem to provide their administrators with any impetus to look further into what they should be trying to accomplish.

"Some departments *spend* money," one high HEW official is supposed to have said. "We just *send* it."

William Gorham, HEW's former assistant secretary, summed up the chaotic situation this way:

We don't have good measures of the effectiveness of most activities in education, health and welfare. . . . We do not follow up graduates of vocational education programs to see how well they do in the labor market. We do not test children from underprivileged homes to find out what kind of school programs work best for them. We do not have records that tell us whether children who go to nursery school do better in subsequent school years or in later life than those who do not.

The federal government is not the only institution that hasn't bothered to evaluate its programs. Our private agencies that purport to "help people" in one way or another have done no better. For years now most of the men who run our private, usually nonprofit social welfare agencies, have been hiding behind the notion that what they do can't be evaluated at all. They have tried to promote the idea that agencies that "help people" produce such intangible results that it is futile to try to judge their success at all. The results of this lethargic attitude are all around us. Our high schools have no idea how many of their graduates remain unemployed or whether their record is better or worse than other high schools. Our hospitals don't know what happens to their patients after they are discharged or even whether they are improved over when they entered. Our welfare agencies don't know how many of their "clients" they have helped obtain better housing or have helped raise out of poverty. In nearly all of our institutions that pride themselves on fashioning a human "product," there is an incredible inertia in approaching what might be called the computation of compassion. An attitude prevails that says, "The business in which we are engaged is so complex that nothing we can measure will adequately portray our effect."

Perhaps not. But because of this attitude it is not so startling that the Defense Department seems to be promoting social progress more rapidly than some of our traditionally more humanistic agencies. In fact, the comparison was not lost on Secretary McNamara himself.

"I am fully aware," he said, "that the Defense Department is not a philanthropic foundation or social welfare institution." But he went on to point out that this fact was no reason to assume that the Defense Department was unable to take steps to alter certain social ills, such as housing discrimination. What's more, the secretary made it perfectly clear that he believed his department could take on such tasks without any jeopardy to its primary goal of national defense. Robert McNamara's attitude was that an immense institution such as the Defense Department can accomplish a diversity of goals—its primary one and many others. "Our primary responsibility . . ." he said, "is the security of this nation. But," he went on, "in the ultimate analysis, the foundation of that security is a stable social structure. I suggest . . . that the Defense Department can find ways to contribute to the development of such a structure. . . ."

In the final analysis, the overriding reason for Mr. McNamara's success in attacking social problems was his determination to do something about them. It was the determination to make a dent in those problems where the efforts of others had failed. It was the determination to confront the housing interests—realtors and landlords—with the facts about how serious the situation really was. It was the determination to act if they proved unable to act. But it was also his determination to attack social problems in a way that would tell him how well he was succeeding that made the difference between the Secretary of Defense and our other officials. Robert McNamara's vision or foresight was no better than that of many other officials. He knew no more about the problems of discrimination in housing, or job training, than many others. But he had the determination and the skill to set up ways of learning about these problems at the same time he was trying to solve them—an accomplishment virtually unparalleled in the federal government.

In so doing he put his fellow officials in other agencies to shame. He made a dent in social problems they'd been fumbling with for years with few tangible results. Furthermore he laid the groundwork for future long-term evaluations of how well his present efforts were working.

The so-called "McNamara method" of solving problems made quite an impression in the government. Other agencies began to try to solve their problems the way he did—or the way they thought he did. They hired scores of systems analysts and operations researchers to help, the same way Mr. McNamara had. They published thick "analyses" of various social problems.

HEW, for instance, began to "analyze" the gamut of social problems, from air pollution to automobile accidents to alcoholism to dozens more. These analyses were supposed to find, in the McNamara jargon, the most "cost-effective" way to cure each of these social ills. The analysis of auto accidents found, for example, that it would cost the government only $87 to save a life by using seat belts, whereas it would cost some $88,000 by using driver education. The cost of providing one classroom seat in an adult education program was found to be $379. The idea of these "analyses" was to decide whether the "benefits" of preventing auto deaths or of providing adult education were worth the costs.

Unfortunately the method soon became the master. HEW's social planners, once again, missed the point. In constructing their analyses, they began to forget about the people whose problems they were supposedly trying to solve. In fact, in adopting the "McNamara method" to the solution of social problems, it almost seems as though the planners soon decided that they couldn't deal with them as people-problems at all and that they would have to treat them as problems that didn't involve people.

In trying to deal with the problem of high school dropouts, for instance, the planners wound up treating the dropout something like a broken piece of machinery. They would simply total up his lifetime earnings and subtract them from the earnings of someone who had finished high school. The

difference represented the "loss" to society. Or to put it another way, the difference was what it would be "worth" to the
government to spend to see that the dropout stayed in school.

The same thing was done for health programs. The lifetime earnings of a forty-five-year-old woman with cancer—
or what it would be "worth" to save her life—were estimated
to be $50,896. The "worth" of a twenty-five-year-old man, on
the other hand—or the "benefit" of saving his life—would be
$128,698.

As the McNamara method gained in vogue, a veritable
deluge of analyses were spewed forth by various government agencies telling what it would be "worth" to improve
people's health, education, and so forth. We can learn by
reading these reports that it would be worthwhile, for instance, to train a man for a new job to the extent that they
will keep earning in a regular and predictable fashion. In
other words, the test of whether or not a particular program
would be worth its cost seemed to be the extent to which the
people who "benefited" would contribute to the Gross
National Product.

An HEW report, for instance, described the results of our
vocational rehabilitation programs in the following way:

> As a result of federal-state vocational rehabilitation
> programs, more than $400 million will be added to the
> nation's personal income next year.

Another federal report talks about the benefits of the Adult
Basic Education Program this way:

> The quantifiable benefits of this program can be
> measured by the anticipated increase in the total life-
> time earnings of the target population. . . .

Another study on the early detection of cancer states that:

> Benefits considered are the estimated savings in earn-
> ing power of . . . persons found with early cancer.

This sort of quasi-humane thinking rapidly became ram-
pant. Scores of federal studies sounded the encouraging note

that "in the long run" it would be more economically bene-
ficial for society to do this or that. This sort of analysis was
usually directed to what needs to be done for poor people,
but not exclusively. We are all, after all, contributors to the
national economy. The best reason our social planners seemed
to say, that could be put forth to justify a program is that it
had a "payoff"—measurable in dollars and cents—greater than
its cost.

Using this reasoning the planners found, for example, that
it was worthwhile to spend money to keep young men in
school instead of paying them to be unemployed. In addition,
they stated (almost apologetically) that staying in school
would somehow be "better for them," though they had little
evidence that it really would be. When the planners wanted
to justify a new health program they used the same reasoning,
merely totaling up the dollars that would be added to the
economy thanks to the illness the new program would, hope-
fully, prevent.

Needless to say, this preoccupation with dollar dividends
from human investment had the danger of obscuring other
gains. It also led to certain embarrassing results in the planners' logic. Since Negroes will not earn as much as whites for
the same amount of schooling, it would obviously make sense
to spend more for schooling whites than Negroes. Since the
aged generally earn nothing, they deserve little or no social
investment at all.

Fortunately our social planners never reached this *reductio
ad absurdum* of "the method." In fact most of the things ad-
vocated because they were found "cost-effective" were also
desirable for other reasons. Job training, preventive health
care, better nutrition, compensatory education—all are usually considered valid goals of an ethically decent society. Yet
it was clear that the planners felt that to "sell these goals to
Congress and the public they must emphasize their economic
benefits—usually in the form of increased earnings for the
persons benefited—rather than any other sorts of less easily
totaled benefits.

Our officials and planners became not advocates but apologists for social decency and concern. They seemed bent on waging war on poverty, not, as Michael Harrington said, because it is "an outrage and a scandal that there should be such social misery," but because it would be economically advantageous—up to a point—to remedy the social needs of the poor than not to.

Much of this sort of thinking was passed off, by our would-be social planners, as the "McNamara method," perhaps because of the former secretary's reputation for cost-saving schemes. But Mr. McNamara, even though he recognized that the Defense Department was not a "social welfare institution," never apologized for his efforts to solve social problems. He never tried to treat human problems as merely economic ones or to tally up the benefits of his programs merely in terms of dollars and cents.

Let us make no mistake. Any way of trying to decide rationally between all the schemes put forth for programs to "improve" people's lives is most likely better than none. Adding up the dollars added to the economy—if these dollars bear any relation to better lives for individuals—is far better than the usual muddleheadedness that prevails when tough choices have to be made. Choices between building more schools or more hospitals. Or between training more teachers versus more doctors. Or between more kidney machines and another moon shot.

But the unabashed glee with which our social welfare came to tout each new program for the megadollars that it would add to our economy is sad testimony to their self-conscious attitude toward noneconomic benefits. It is a sad commentary on their apologetic attitude toward improving human capabilities and aspirations—the sort of attitude that says, "We ought to do such-and-such because it will add to our national productivity and, by the way, will also make people less miserable."

This new sort of quasi-humanism scarcely gets us any closer toward finding out how our society can improve its performance in fostering social progress. It doesn't tell us anything about in what areas we are now failing to do as well as we could in bettering people's lives. In fact it only feeds the fires of those people who like to mutter complacently that social progress can't be dealt with methodically— the same sort of people who believe that in some strange way the Social Security System's computers are destroying our freedom or that some nebulous "personal" element is being lost.

It is hard to say which brand of thinking is more dangerous—the kind that reduces human values to economic ones or the kind that believes that there is a menace in treating social problems precisely and systematically. Fortunately, however, most Americans aren't afraid of having their problems dealt with in the latter fashion. Nearly everyone would prefer to receive a computer-sent monthly Social Security check than be visited each month by a friendly social worker who would personally determine how much money he needs for food, shoes, and so forth. Most people would prefer to receive a computer-sent Medicare check than be interviewed by a hospital official to find out whether they can afford care for a heart attack. Ask your neighbor whether he'd rather some distant computer sent him a card entitling his daughter to free school lunches because she was underweight and poor or whether he'd rather be paid a visit by his friendly local Agricultural Extension agent.

We could use a dose of compassion in this country—the logical, systematic, precise kind of compassion that emanates from the well-programmed computer and not from capricious local, state, or even federal officials. The computation of compassion is something we need more of, not less.

We've seen how haphazardly most of our institutions that do "good works" are run—including the federal government. Most in fact don't even know how haphazardly they are run because they've never kept the records by which it would be possible to find out. Our schools know what they spend for each student but not what it costs to teach a child to read. Our hospitals have no idea whether it costs them more to perform brain surgery or to take someone's tonsils out. Our public agencies don't know how much their programs cost or who benefits from them. These institutions are still trying to hoist themselves into the twentieth century. They are trying to get used to the idea that there is an efficient and effective way to teach someone to read or to take out an appendix, or to train a drill press operator. Once the folks who run these agencies rid themselves of the notion that they deserve credit for merely doing good works regardless of how well or efficiently they do them, then we can begin to look forward to a more rational sort of compassion. Then, and only then, can we afford to smirk at the idea that the Defense Department may be contributing more to social progress than any other public or private institution.

The federal government jumped into the computation of compassion with both feet. There was a giant splash—but little else. Robert McNamara was doubtless amused by some of the elaborate analyses of social problems that masqueraded under the name of the "McNamara method." But Mr. McNamara would also probably be the first to agree that very little in these analyses will advance our overall rate of social progress until their authors begin to treat the solutions to social problems as ones whose benefits add up to more than the economic ones we are able to measure so well.

# CHAPTER
# 9

## Measuring the Rate of Social Progress

There is a large windowless storeroom on the top floor of the Department of Health, Education and Welfare building in Washington where copies of various government reports are kept. The last time I was there several large cartons occupied one corner of the room. Inside each carton were dozens of copies of a document as thick as the Manhattan telephone directory. At the top of its powder-blue cover, in brown letters, were the words "Administrative Confidential—Not for Quoting." Then, in larger print, the title: *Materials for Preliminary Draft of the Social Report*.

Some of the cartons were half empty. Most had never even been opened. I dug into one open carton, and stuck a copy of the heavy book under one arm. One of the file clerks looked up casually.

"Take all you want," she said. "Take them all."

I still have my copy. Someday it may well be a historic document—this bulky mimeographed volume bound with an aluminum strip, all its chapters in different type, some of its numerous tables and graphs so poorly reproduced as to be nearly illegible—for this volume was the promising start of one of the least publicized, but most ambitious and energetic social projects ever initiated by the federal government. It was a project that lasted more than two years and eventually came to involve dozens of consultants and staff personnel. This undertaking was nothing less than the serious attempt on the part of the federal government to measure the nation's rate of social progress.

On March 1, 1966, President Johnson in a little-noticed paragraph of one of his annual messages to Congress issued a directive to the Secretary of Health, Education and Welfare.

"To improve our ability to chart our progress," the President's message said,

> I have asked the Secretary to establish within his office the resources to develop the necessary social statistics and indicators to supplement those prepared by the Bureau of Labor Statistics and the Council of Economic Advisors.

"With these yardsticks," the directive concluded, "we can better measure the distance we have come and plan for the way ahead."

The President's directive met with many reactions. The development of additional statistics with which to measure social progress clearly signified different things to different people. To some it raised the spectre of an ever-curious government prying into citizens' private lives—a government for whom more complete information on the life styles of Americans presaged the possible attempt at more stringent control of these life styles. The fact that this information was to be gathered by a "social" agency such as HEW did not assuage the suspicions of those who feared the government's motives.

"It's a race between the do-gooders and the police," one Washingtonian told me, "to see who will develop the first complete dossier on everyone."

There may have been more than a grain of truth in the suspicion that the collection of "necessary social statistics and indicators" was not ordered with completely altruistic motives in mind. A good deal of support for better "indicators" of social progress and change came from federal officials concerned about how to prevent riots and other civil disturbances. A book entitled *Social Indicators*, written under a contract with NASA as a discussion of the social effects of the space program, used crime rates as an example of a social "indicator." There was a strong feeling among some officials that, with more complete social data, civil disorders could be more easily headed off. There was even talk of constructing a "riot index" of all the major American cities, using data on unemployment, population density, crime rates, and a host of other information in the government's files. The most Machiavellian of planners actually believed that accurate prediction of a city's riot "threshold" by the use of various statistical measures would enable the federal or local government to redirect social programs into such an area, thus reducing the boiling point. This sort of "fireplug mentality," as when local officials put sprinklers on fire plugs to cool off ghetto children during the summer, had many adherents in the government.

Another more constructive reaction to the President's directive came from those individuals with genuine interest in social problems and policies. Most of these observers, both inside and outside the government, felt the kind of effort mandated by the directive was long overdue. They considered the traditional economic indicators of social progress—those indicators which had been developed in response to the Employment Act of 1946—to be necessary but hardly sufficient for an adequate picture of national social progress. Why, many asked, shouldn't the nation know at least as much —in an objective way—about the growth of social opportunity and equality as we now know about the growth of the Gross National Product? Why should we not know as much about how well our schoolchildren are learning to read this year or about how healthy our people are or about how much job opportunity exists or about numerous other social facts as we know about how many freight cars are loaded each month or how many tons of steel are produced?

Many even argued that there should be a national social report that would, in a fashion analogous to the annual Economic Report mandated by the Employment Act, present a yearly accounting of the social status of the nation.

It was with this end in mind—the publication of the nation's first social report—that the Department of Health, Education and Welfare under Secretary John Gardner began to respond to the presidential directive. A staff was hastily assembled. Consultants from universities and "think tanks" were flown to Washington for meetings. A panel of consultants headed by Daniel Bell, a Columbia University sociologist, and William Gorham, one of Mr. Gardner's assistant secretaries who had joined HEW after working as a systems analyst for Robert McNamara at the Pentagon, was established to give direction to the enterprise.

At the outset Gorham and Bell in a confidential memorandum to the entire panel broached the task in challenging terms.

"No society in history," they said, "has, as yet, made a coherent and unified effort to assess those elements . . . which bar each individual from realizing to the fullest extent possible his talents and abilities. . . ." No nation, in other words, had ever published a social report.

Mr. Gorham, for one, was optimistic about the panel's early progress. In July of 1967 he testified before a Senate subcommittee as follows:

> The panel is off to a promising start. Some sections of the Report—particularly those on opportunity and on the quality of the environment—have been extensively outlined. Others are in less formative stages with conceptual problems still unresolved.

Several months later Mr. Gorham was still optimistic. "Our work," he said,

> on social indicators has been under way for about a year and has enlisted the support of our most distinquished social scientists. It is too soon to report substantive findings but I can convey to you the guarded optimism of a number of our government and academic skeptics.

Outside the federal government, as Mr. Gorham had said, confidence was high that the nation's first social report would soon be finished. Bertram Gross, one of the strong proponents of the idea, in the *Annals of the Academy of Political and Social Sciences*, predicted that "the President may soon initiate a series of annual social reports to Congress. This could be done without new legislative authority."

No doubt at that time Dr. Gross felt that the possibility of a soon-to-be-released social report was very likely. A few months later it seemed even more likely. The cardboard boxes on the fifth floor of HEW were crammed with the report's thick preliminary drafts. The chapters had engaging titles compared to those of most government reports: Health and Life; Opportunity; Learning, Science and Culture; Race Relations and Social Change. Each chapter was supposed to present certain "social indicators" concerning the area under discussion and draw conclusions from these indicators about the amount of social progress that had occurred and the amount that was possible in the near future. In addition, each chapter was to suggest new ways of measuring progress —the new "indicators" President Johnson had requested in his directive.

Soon after the draft had been finished, however, the ambitious undertaking ran into trouble. Various task forces were formed, each of which was supposed to have the responsibility for reviewing a different chapter. These task forces were composed, for the most part, of consultants the government had hired, mainly people from the so-called academic community.

I remember attending an early meeting of the health task force. The chairman was a hard-faced woman, an executive of a New York foundation. She began by berating the HEW staff members who had prepared a draft of the chapter on health for the task force. She called the draft totally inadequate. She acted as though the government were insulting her by paying her plane fare to Washington to read such a shoddy piece of work. Then she and the other members settled into a discussion of how best to measure the nation's health. Someone would suggest a particular measure and the others would disagree. When the afternoon was over the group had not been able to agree on a single valid measure for the nation's health. They adjourned, presumably to fly back to their various foundations and universities, having agreed only that the measurement of the nation's health was difficult indeed and that none of the present statistics were adequate.

Needless to say the government's consultants, for the most part, were of little help in the writing of the social report. If —as I mentioned to one of my co-workers—the health task force could not agree on any decent measures of the nation's health, I wondered what hope there was that the other task forces would agree on ways to measure less tangible things. What chances, I wondered, would there be that they could agree on how best to measure such phenomena as social opportunity or participation.

The forthcoming social report ran into other difficulties as well. There was trouble obtaining skilled staff members to work on the report. Most HEW officials had no interest in the social report whatsoever. There were too many other things to do, they thought, than waste time writing a report on the social state of the nation. Many looked upon the report as just another chore—something Secretary Gardner was doing in order to give HEW academic prestige. These officials resented being asked to leave their regular jobs, even for a short while, to help on the report. To make matters worse, those who did help resented the numerous well-paid consultants who flew to Washington periodically, told them they were doing an inadequate job of writing the report, and then flew back home without offering any constructive suggestions.

Virtually all the HEW officials who helped in writing the report were ordered to do so. There were practically no volunteers from within HEW for the task of trying to measure the nation's social progress. I remember one middle-aged woman statistician who was working on the report. She had been "detailed"—against her will, she said—from her regular job and was supposed to pick up the writing of one of the chapters where another disgruntled staff member, who had just quit, had left off.

"I don't know the first thing about most of this stuff," she confided. "This has nothing to do with my specialty. They just put me in this office with all these materials," pointing to a huge stack of papers and books, "and told me to start writing." She threw up her hands in a gesture of despair.

"I can't wait to get out of here," she said.

The whole thing—a frail woman statistician held captive and told to write part of a social report—would be funny, like some sort of fairy tale, if it had not been so true. It would be humorous were it not for the many people who were forced, with little interest and in many cases with no appropriate skill, to help write the report.

In January, 1969, what was supposed to be the social report was finally published. However it was not a social report as its title "Toward a Social Report" clearly indicated. After more than two years of effort, with the support of some of our most distinguished social scientists, the several-hundred-page preliminary draft of the report had shrunk to a pamphlet of barely a hundred pages that did not purport to be a report on the social state of the nation at all. The new "report's" introduction, in fact, made this quite clear:

> The present report is not a social report. It is a step in
> the direction of a social report and the development
> of a comprehensive set of social indicators.

In his letter transmitting the report to President Johnson, HEW's new secretary, Wilbur Cohen, called the document a "preliminary step" that "paves the way" for a real full-fledged social report. He believed, Mr. Cohen told the President, that thanks to "the preliminary steps already developed under your leadership . . . a first social report could be developed within two years."

This thin report was considerably different from the original powder-blue draft stacked in HEW's top-floor closet. It was, in fact, a considerably watered-down version of the original draft. The new report, for instance, omitted the chapter "Race Relations and Social Change." This chapter had begun by listing "the general areas in which Negroes currently experience a deficit compared to other Americans." These areas were described in the chapter as "areas of desired social change." The chapter then went on to describe ways in which these Negro deficits could be "converted" to assets. This chapter, in its author's words, described how "a distinct subgroup, in society, without power and without the direct resources for gaining power, can nevertheless come to gain power . . . the power of each individual implied in a document like the Constitution."

Several other portions of the original draft had also disappeared from the final report. The original draft had contained a lengthy section devoted to the legal rights of poor Americans. This section discussed the failure of our legal system to adequately represent and defend the poor, and it presented data to support this claim. "There is good reason to believe," this section noted, "that the very persons who would benefit most by the exercise of rights of appeal do so least." The final report, however, contained none of these facts.

Instead it contained three short paragraphs on justice in the courts, commenting finally that "it is extremely difficult to collect information on shortcomings. . . ."

The original draft contained a long section on man's environment. It contained a list of possible goals for the reduction of various air pollutants. It contained a table showing the levels of water pollution in various United States rivers. The final draft devoted four pages to these problems. It contained no air pollution goals or water pollution levels. It told the reader only that a major reduction in air pollution "will not be easy" and made a similar pessimistic statement about water pollution.

The original draft contained many pages of information on whether or not Americans were healthier, better-educated, or had more opportunity than, let us say, a decade ago—but the final report contained practically none of this information.

The final report had become little more than a collection of stale clichés. "The greatest challenge to American education," the final report said, ". . . is to find effective ways of helping low-income children learn the basic intellectual skills so that they can be more successful in school and compete more successfully for jobs and rewarding positions in the community. . . ."

The final report contained this comment on the role of science in society:

> The benefits of basic research are international, and worldwide cooperation in science is essential. A cooperative recognition of the universality of basic science could benefit all mankind.

It said this about the problem of crowding in our urban ghettos:

> It is not possible to say for certain whether such crowding degrades the quality of life significantly for very many people. . . . It is evident from any number

2

t46

---

of parks and beaches that, just as a few seek secluded spots, so many others congregate wherever the most people are.

The final report made no effort to develop any new measures of social progress as President Johnson had requested two years earlier. The report made virtually no effort to pinpoint the areas in which the nation could be making more rapid social progress.

The report was not, of course, totally worthless. It made, at least, an attempt—as its authors said—to "pose important questions." It made an attempt to point out how little was known about how slowly or rapidly the nation was making social progress. The report pointed out that despite the fact that the government employed almost 19,000 statistical workers and spent 88 million dollars in 1967, only "a small fraction of the existing statistics tell us anything about social conditions. . . ."

The report also pointed out certain things that other government reports had not emphasized. It pointed out that there was probably no more opportunity in America now than existed ten or even twenty years ago. It brought to light a government survey *done in 1962* that had shown that most Negro men, regardless of their father's occupations, were working at unskilled or semiskilled jobs. The report dredged up previously unpublished data—more than six years old—to show that, at least in 1962, social opportunity was still seriously limited by race.

The report found unpublished data from a three-year-old survey of educational opportunity done by the government's Office of Education that showed that one-half of all high school graduates who rank in the top 20 percent of their class —if their parents come from the "bottom socioeconomic quartile"—will not go to college.

The report, in other words, pointed out some things that other government reports should have emphasized long ago. But clearly, in terms of the early ambitions of Assistant Secretary Gorham and others, the report that finally was issued was hardly what had been planned.

"The mountain labored," one experienced official said, "and gave birth to a mouse."

What was the point of trying to measure national social progress at all? We are already glutted with information on society's ills and on what is being done to combat them. We already have books on every conceivable social problem. Our newspapers tell us what is being done to solve these problems. Our federal government collects massive amounts of statistics each year—statistics on every aspect of human life—statistics that tell how long it's been since you last visited a dentist or how many micrograms of DDT are in your daily milk. Data on everything from pollution in the ionosphere to pollution in uranium mines. Everyone knows, we might suppose—if they want to know—about these problems and how fast we're moving to solve them.

Americans, so the story goes, have always been aware of the importance of progress. "Progress is our most important product," says Madison Avenue. Every year new stories of progress fill our yearbooks—a new vaccine, a new supersonic plane, a new desalinization process, or a new photographic emulsion. We are told that the breakneck pace of progress is almost more than the nation can tolerate. Everyone, we are told, is in most ways better off than ever before. The average American earns more money, purchases more, eats a better diet, and has taller children. Most Americans have sincerely believed that progress is both inevitable and is occurring at an ever accelerating rate.

A few have not. In his book *Teaching the "Unteachable"* Herbert Kohl wrote, "I had been assigned to teach . . . an unreal myth about a country that has never existed. I didn't believe the tale of 'progress' the curriculum had prescribed."

Government reports usually present a particularly euphoric picture of social progress. After the summer riots of 1967, for instance, President Johnson requested that government statisticians prepare an official report on the status of Negro

Americans. This report was to present a "balanced picture" of Negro progress—a picture based on "facts."

"These facts," said the report, when it appeared, "show a mixture of sound and substantial progress, on the one hand, and large unfilled needs on the other." A safe enough statement for a government report—a statement designed to please everyone.

Was the report right? Did the "facts" it presented—and those it did not—demonstrate any "sound and substantial progress"?

Most of the report made no effort to assess the social progress of the Negro at all. In some strange way the assessment of Negro progress became transformed into an assessment of economic progress, complete with the same economic statistics and clichés that had been used in government reports for years. Here is how the report summarized the progress of Negro Americans:

> The single most important fact in the economic life of most Americans—white and Negro alike—is the great productivity of our economy. . . . The incomes of both whites and Negroes are at an all time high and during the last year the gap between the two has significantly narrowed. . , . Unemployment rates for nonwhites are still twice those for whites, but the level for both groups has dropped dramatically. . . . Education has often been considered the key to economic success. . . . Recent improvements for nonwhites . . . parallel those previously described in employment and income. . . .

Somehow the "economic life" of Americans seemed to be all that really mattered to the government's report writers, for most of their report was devoted to economic "indicators" of progress. Unfortunately, however, even this simpleminded way of looking at progress didn't prove that any progress had actually occurred!

The report stated that the income gap between whites and

"nonwhites" had "significantly narrowed" in the last year. This "fact" was presented as the first proof of progress. What the report failed to emphasize, however, was the fact that during the previous year the income gap between whites and nonwhites actually increased—a curious sort of sustained progress indeed. Furthermore a Harvard professor, Lester Thurow, gave another less optimistic picture of how rapidly the incomes of different groups of Americans were becoming more equal at a congressional hearing:

> When we look at the income distribution, there have been no changes in the postwar period. In relative terms the gap between rich and poor has remained constant. . . . There is no evidence that the income distribution is becoming more equal, either between rich and poor, or between black and white.

"In terms of their income distribution," Professor Thurow told Congress, "the nonwhite population is lagging approximately thirty years behind the white. . . . This was true in 1947. It is true in 1966."

In other words there were still as many Americans, relatively speaking, at the bottom of the economic heap as there were in 1947. What's more, they were probably the same Americans or their descendants.

The government report on the status of Negro Americans exulted over the progress made in eradicating Negro unemployment. The level of unemployment, for white and nonwhites, has "dropped dramatically," the report said. But there was another side. Senator William Proxmire had said on the same subject at a recent hearing that the rise in nonwhite unemployment from 5.9 to 7.4 percent over the twenty-year period since the Employment Act was made law "does not suggest to me" that opportunities for Negroes to work have improved. An NAACP statement on job opportunity also did not quite square with the government report's optimism. "Given a continuation of the present rates of advance," said the NAACP, "it will take Negroes 138 years, or until

2094 to secure equal participation in skilled, craft training and employment."

What about education? In this area, said the report, "Improvements . . . paralleled those in employment and income." For once the report was right. Improvements in education had paralleled those in employment and income—that is, they had been just as imaginary. But this is evidently not what the authors of the report meant. Listen to their enthusiastic rhetoric on the subject of Negro education:

> Many Negroes have taken advantage of education and training programs in recent years. The fact that these opportunities exist, and that large numbers of Negroes are using them, proves that there are open avenues of upward mobility in our society. Many who were at the bottom are finding their way up the economic ladder.

"We will stand on that," said the authors.

Perhaps a rather daring statement to stand upon, especially since the report's authors could produce no figures that would give any idea just how many Negroes "at the bottom" were climbing their way up that lyrical socioeconomic ladder.

The report's statistics had very little relevance to economic, let alone social, progress for Negroes. The report said that "over 28 percent of . . . nonwhite families received more than $7,000 a year—more than double the proportion with incomes that high seven years ago." Is this a meaningful statement? Does it mean that nonwhite families are improving their incomes at a satisfactory pace as compared with other families? The authors of the report offered no comment on this score although they must have known that, in Professor Thurow's words, "measures of income dispersion indicate no progress to a more egalitarian income distribution since World War II."

To make matters worse, here is how the authors of this report replied when they were severely criticized for failing to consider what, if anything, their statistics meant or "proved":

> We were not asked for . . . technical analysis . . . we were not asked for a learned essay concerning the failings of social statistics. . . . The aim was to present an objective view of the situation of Negroes in America based on facts so that a troubled nation could turn to facts for guidance. . . .

"We were not asked for a monograph intended for specialists," the authors said in further defense of their report. One can only wonder, if they had been so asked, whether they could have produced such a monograph. One wonders if they would even agree that Americans are entitled to, if not a monograph, at least a meaningful analysis of the situation.

Apparently these report writers had confused "facts" with figures. They had apparently confused "an objective view of the situation" with an unthinking and uncritical one. In other words, like most of our would-be experts, they purported to just present the "facts" when what they were really doing was avoiding any critical thought about what their "facts" signified or how pertinent they were to the issue at hand. Moreover some facts were entirely left out of the report.

The report's writers chose not to emphasize, for example—as the Violence Commission later pointed out—the fact that black men in cities who worked the year round earned about seven-tenths as much as white workers, and that "this fraction was unchanged since 1959."

The report's authors might also have estimated with a fair degree of accuracy just how much of the income gap between whites and "nonwhites" was due to differences in educational or occupational levels as opposed to racial discrimination. Data existed in government files to make this sort of estimate. Data existed to judge whether that part of the gap due to discrimination was changing for the better or not. The report's authors could have examined the several studies that had been done on the subject of American social mobility to try to see if Negroes who were at the bottom of the heap a few years ago were truly any better off today. There is no hint, however, that our "objective" experts thought to look at this information, much of it gathered with the help of government funds, and available in the government's files.

The report's writers ignored these and many other sources of relevant information and instead relied upon "facts" that did not go very far toward portraying that picture of "widespread . . . social and economic gains experienced by most Negroes in recent years." Rashi Fein and Stephen Michelson, two economists at Washington's Brookings Institution, hit the nail on the head when they noted that this song has become a broken record for Americans. A government report on "The Economic and Social Progress of the Negro Population," *published in 1918*, pointed out Fein and Michelson, said exactly the same thing! As the two economists put it:

> . . . for 50 years government studies have concluded that the Negro is making substantial progress, that he has not yet achieved equality, that we should not be pessimistic, but that we dare not be complacent.

The government's hurriedly produced report on the status of Negro Americans is a good example of why something better—an annual, candid assessment of social progress—is needed. The government's report, indeed, hardly stressed *social* progress at all, but rather "the great productivity of our economy."

Can this nation—or any nation—actually determine how rapidly it is making social progress or how fast it is enhancing the opportunities or aspirations of its people? Can the nation say whether or not, as an entire society, it is performing to full capacity in bettering the lives of all its citizens? The writing of the nation's first social report was begun with these questions in mind. The report was to be a national social balance sheet—a record of the gains and losses, the credits and debits in our year-by-year struggle for social progress. It was to point out serious or worsening social problems as well as those for which progress had been made. It was to inform Americans of those areas where the nation could be making progress more rapidly—those areas of unfulfilled national potential.

Why was the report never completed? Why was the job of telling Americans how well we are doing and how well we might be doing curtailed? Was the social report just a utopian dream—an unrealistic, idealistic hope of spinning tales of social progress sprung full-blown from the brains of Washington bureaucrats? Was it just another political maneuver to convince the nation that, indeed, something was being done—or was going to be done—about the nation's pressing social problems?

Perhaps the social report was never completed because the task was too big. Perhaps the experts and officials had bitten off more than they could chew. But there is another possibility too. Perhaps the unfinished report's would-be authors discovered, in attempting to assess the nation's recent social progress, that when the trouble was taken to look honestly at the situation very little evidence of recent social progress could be found.

Reading the original draft of the social report—that thick tome stacked in HEW's storeroom—this is exactly the impression one gains: that very little objective proof of recent social progress could be mustered. The draft's chapter on health, for example, pointed out that the "length of life for the American people has not increased appreciably since 1950"— despite continued progress in other nations. The death rate in New York City was actually higher in 1968 than in 1945; infant death rates were higher than fifteen years ago. Deaths of mothers in childbirth were nearly 50 percent higher than the year before. A black infant, born in one of our nation's ghettos, has no better chance of reaching his first birthday, compared to his white neighbor, than he did ten years ago.

In some cities his chances are actually *worse* than a decade ago.

In education the story is similar. There has been a gradual but definite slowdown in our capability to educate our people. Youngsters obtain essentially no more years of schooling now than they did five years ago. As the original draft of the social report pointed out, between 1955 and 1965 the percentage of male high school graduates who went to college actually decreased. Negro students in New York City, says Kenneth Clark, actually learned *more*, compared with whites, in 1930 than they do today. As the draft of the social report also pointed out, the chances of a talented high school student from a poverty family getting into a four-year college, compared with those of his well-to-do classmates, were no better in 1960, when the government last looked into the matter, than they were twenty years earlier. In another fifteen years, if present trends continue, we still won't be anywhere near equality of educational opportunity: by 1985 enough Negroes still won't have been admitted to college, or even have finished high school, to assure them a chance of making an income comparable to that of whites even assuming discrimination did not exist.

There is no evidence that job discrimination has decreased markedly in the last decade. Some studies in fact state that it has increased. Compared to whites, nonwhites stood a better chance of being employed ten years ago than they do today! The original draft of the social report, in fact, said exactly this: that there was no evidence for an appreciable decrease in job discrimination in the last ten years.

Segregation in housing has—to all appearances—remained essentially at the same level as in 1958. The draft of the social report noted that in six major American cities for which data were available housing segregation was no less than in 1960. In fact in five of the six it had increased. And there was no reason to think the story was not similar in other major cities.

The government's studies of family diets, as well as other

evidence, suggests that the nutrition of Americans may be no better now than in 1955. "Malnutrition among the poor," said the Citizens' Board of Inquiry, "has risen sharply over the past decade."

The original draft of the social report was not a sugar-coated document. It pointed out, in each of these areas and in many others, how little social progress could be seen. It set forth, also, many areas in which there was evidence that the nation was doing better now than, let us say, ten years ago. It set forth, in other words, both the credits and the debits. But, as so often happens, the latter were largely forgotten in the government's final version of the report.

There may have been still another reason it was decided not to publish the original social report. The writers of the unfinished social report found, in addition to the fact that not much social progress was demonstrable, that not much was known about social problems in general. All in all they found our ignorance about the nation's social problems—despite the millions of dollars our government spends to find out—is amazing.

Have our lives really changed for the better? Are we really better off than ten years ago? Have we given *all* our citizens a chance for a better life? Does a black man or a poor man have a better chance of buying a home of his choice, compared to his next-door neighbor who is neither black nor poor, than a decade ago? No one can really answer questions such as these. Not because they have no answers, but simply because we have never taken the trouble to look for them. As a nation we have never really faced up to the questions themselves.

"The nation has no comprehensive set of statistics," said the final report, "reflecting social progress or retrogression.

"If a balanced, organized, and concise set of measures of the condition of our society were available," the report stated, "we should have the information needed to identify emerging problems and to make knowledgeable decisions about national priorities."

The last nationwide survey of overcrowded housing was in 1960. Many of our cities have no idea how much of their housing is dilapidated or overcrowded. They have no idea how many people live in this sort of housing or how long they have been living there.

There has never been a nationwide survey of educational achievement. When the government tried to check on the success of its teaching programs for disadvantaged children, less than half the nation's one hundred largest school systems could supply the necessary facts. Virtually none of our school systems have followed its children from grade to grade, checking their learning each year. The last national survey showing how many high school students go on to college was in 1960.

We have only just begun a national nutrition survey. We can only guess at the number of malnourished Americans. There has never been a national health survey that can tell us how one city compares to another. Minneapolis can't even guess whether the health of its people is improving faster than that of folks across the river in St. Paul.

There has never been a national inventory of the sources of water pollution.

What are some of the reasons for our overwhelming ignorance about not only the magnitude of our social problems, but also about where they are worst or are getting worse?

Social progress has always been regarded as something that was, if not inevitable, at least part and parcel of overall economic progress. It has always been thought of as something that may be facilitated by our massive social programs, but not—unlike economic progress—very susceptible to control. It was never thought conceivable that such measures of social progress as infant mortality rates, high school reading levels, juvenile delinquency rates, and a variety of measures of social dependency could be altered in a desired way by appropriate decisions. It was never thought possible that the life expectancy of Americans might be no less a social policy decision than their unemployment rate. For this reason social progress—both for individuals and the nation as a whole—has never had its "bill of rights" that guarantees all citizens the basic requirements for human growth and development. There are no national goals to assure these rights. There is no goal that every child should have a yearly doctor's visit. Or that he should be entitled to a year's worth of learning for every year spent in school. Or that he should be entitled to grow up in an uncrowded, safe environment. There is no national goal that says that his father should have the opportunity to advance, according to ability, in his line of work. Or that he should be able to change jobs easily. Or that his mother should have health care during her next pregnancy or day care for her preschool children. There is no national goal that assures Americans the right to participate to the fullest in the decisions of their society or its institutions.

Economic progress, on the other hand, has had its goals laid out for some twenty years. The Employment Act of 1946 stated three goals of economic well-being: full employment; economic growth; and stable prices. These were the three indices by which the nation agreed to try to measure economic "success." Since 1946 their measurement and interpretation has been largely the job of the Council of Economic Advisors. Needless to say, these goals are also "social" ones. Full employment is as much a social goal as an economic one. But the fact remains that the reason we measure employment is as an index of economic well-being, not human well-being.

The proof of this is simply that, since the Employment Act, we have learned to measure economic progress in detail and with a precision no less than amazing, while, at the same time, our measurement of social progress has been practically nonexistent. We know a great deal about investment in factories and equipment, but very little about investment in humans. The economist can follow a pound of iron ore from the mine to its place in your television tube, but we don't know how many high school graduates go on to college each year. We know quite precisely how fast our factories are becoming outmoded, but not how fast our job skills are. We know infinitely more about new housing starts or freight-car loadings than new career starts. Our economists can tell us the costs of manufacturing an extra television set but not of taking out an appendix.

It is only recently that a few Americans are starting to realize that there is more to running a successful society than a rising GNP or more freight-car loadings. Some people have begun to ask why we can make more than enough miles of pipe and yet lack plumbing in thousands of American homes. They ask why can we make more than enough washing machines and yet lack the artificial kidneys to wash the poisons out of 3,600 people who die each year. Some Americans are beginning to wonder why we seem to be able to teach our soldiers Laotian in six months, but can't teach our schoolchildren English in twelve years. Or why we can rescue wounded men in Vietnam in a matter of minutes, but accident victims lie on our highways for hours. Many people are beginning to ask just what rate of "deliberate social change," to use a phrase coined by Anatole Rapoport, they have a right to expect from the world's richest nation. They are asking why a nation that could anticipate postwar recession, and take steps to guarantee economic progress, cannot do the same for its citizens' social needs.

It is obviously easier to assess the economic progress of a nation than it is to measure its social progress. There is no good way to measure the dull look of futility in the eyes of Jonathan Kozol's schoolchildren—though we know that it exists. There is no way to measure the exhaustion of a mother who has waited all day in the clinic of an urban hospital—though we know it is real. There is no way to measure the conviction of a high school dropout that staying in school will not help him get a better job—but it is present all the same. These things—hopes, feelings, human energy—are important in our equation for social progress. Unfortunately, or perhaps fortunately, we cannot measure them. Actually it is more accurate to say that we have never really tried.

The more we do start to measure, however, the more a disturbing picture emerges. A picture of a nation where social progress can hardly be taken for granted, where many of our people are actually becoming worse off while others improve. A nation where the gaps between rich and poor, black and white, are not always diminishing and in some ways are yawning wider every year. One by one the myths about America's progress that we have been brought up to believe are being laid to rest. America is not now it seems likely—any more than a decade ago—the land of opportunity. It is not the land of greater freedom from hunger and want. It is not the land of more justice for all. All its children are not better educated nor healthier. In practically every area of human concern, wherever someone has taken the trouble to look carefully at the trends, the same story has emerged.

And what we know is only the tip of the iceberg. As a nation and a society we have never really bothered to gather the simple facts to assess our performance in improving people's lives. There is hardly a single social problem for which anything more than the scantiest information is available to answer the question: "Are we doing better this year than last year or than ten years ago?"

Our experts have few of the answers. They too suffer from the same lack of relevant facts, though they possess a plethora of irrelevant ones. If you ask a school superintendent how well his school is performing, he will most likely tell you how many teachers he employs who have advanced teaching degrees or what the size of his classrooms are—not what his pupils are learning or how many of them get jobs after graduation. If you ask a hospital administrator how good his hospital is, he will probably say "Well you know we have Dr. So-and-so, the world's greatest kidney surgeon," or he will tell you how many people were seen in the clinic last year. In all those areas where experts have held sway, more often that not what they have tried to pass off as progress have been merely the "inputs" to progress.

Whether, in fact, progress has occurred is anyone's conjecture. In most ways, on a nationwide scale, we have very little idea whether we are doing better or worse than a decade ago. Do our children read better, across the country, than they did in 1960? Do they eat better? Do they have less tooth decay? Are our young men more physically fit? Are less people living in overcrowded housing?

As Mr. Gorham put it:

> In health we have plentiful statistics on mortality and morbidity but almost nothing which will tell us whether people are significantly healthier than they used to be. In education we know a great deal about the resources used to teach children, but almost nothing about what is accomplished. Do children in fact learn more now than they used to? We think so, but we have no way to know.

Americans are starting to realize that all too often progress in these areas has nothing to do with the volumes of statistics that pour daily from a thousand government agencies and bureaus. These statistics rarely measure opportunity. They practically never measure equality. Is it important that so many thousand units of housing were built last year if we cannot say whether more people can buy decent housing at a reasonable price or in the neighborhood of their choice? Does it matter that we can transplant a heart if we do not know how many children never get to see a dentist? Does it matter if the average family income doubles if most families are still where they were in 1947—no better, no worse? Our statistics never measure aspiration. How many high school seniors want to go to college but can't find a place? How many mothers want remedial reading or day-care services for their children but can't find them? How many adults want job training but can't obtain it?

There is no Gross National Product for human growth. There is no computer in Washington that tallies the daily gain or loss in human potential. There is no meter that registers the waste of human energy. Millions of children sit impassively in school each day while their intellects are destroyed and their energy to learn is melted away, but not a page in the government's statistical abstracts tells of this loss.

The nation's first social report is still unfinished. The last time I bothered to look, the cartons filled with its preliminary drafts were still stacked in their Washington closet. They are probably still in the same place. Whether anyone is interested in finishing the report is questionable. But of one thing we can be certain—the nation needs such an accounting and needs it now more than ever before.

# CHAPTER
## 10

# *The Satisficers*

The day after the Washington riots began, I visited the woman physician with whom I had worked the night before trying to help the riot victims. We ate lunch in her tiny office on HEW's top floor. The smell of smoldering ruins hung over the city. Washington was under martial law. Everywhere one could see guardsmen sitting atop their jeeps, bayonets pointing skyward.

The walls of the office were bare, save for a small card pasted over the desk. On it was typed a single sentence: "The good is the enemy of the best."

I asked her about this aphorism.

"It's from Voltaire, I think," she said, with a smile. "I don't even know if that's really what he said. I keep it there to remind me every time I'm tempted to settle for doing a job that is only good enough. It's my reminder not to satisfice."

Unfortunately, not everyone working in the government shared her attitude. Many, in fact, saw their entire existence as a struggle to get by with doing a job that was just good enough.

"Just remember one thing," one official told me when I first came to Washington. "Whenever anyone asks you to prepare a report or to answer an inquiry or to do anything, the first rule is to satisfice."

I often thought of all the tasks that I had seen—during my short stay in Washington—satisficed by federal officials. Difficult tasks such as the one involving the kidney machine, where, instead of putting in the difficult work and coming up with even a partial solution, the whole issue had been purposely muddled and confused. Problems of child health care, where the officials charged with running this program seemed to think it would satisfice to pass a new law without doing anything new about the problem.

There were problems like the Pennsylvania man's complaint, where merely conducting an investigation seemed to be all the bureaucrats thought they needed to do to satisfice. Or the problem posed by the Poor People's Campaign, where the way to satisfice seemed to be to promise dozens of conferences, reports, and studies, without ever actually doing anything. There were problems like those of hunger and malnutrition, where it seemed adequate to simply overlook the whole situation while reassuring the public that there was really no problem at all.

There were larger problems like planning social programs or trying to see whether or not they were working, problems where what our officials thought was a good enough job would, I felt certain, not be good enough for most American taxpayers. And there was the social report, what was supposed to be a complete status report on the social state of the nation, but which turned into something called "Toward a Social Report"—a pamphlet whose very title was a perfect example of satisficing.

The satisficers seemed to be everywhere, and they seemed to always want to convince others that things were going "well enough" already. Their attitude was always "don't make waves," "don't rock the boat."

I recall one government adviser, a well-known political scientist, who was asked to comment on a special report to be sent to President Johson which recommended a major reorganization of HEW. The adviser's attitude was a typical one.

"Perhaps we have . . . a fundamental difference of opinion," he stated, "as to whether we are serving either the President or the department well, by the emphasis these pages put on the need for coordinating social programs."

The adviser, hired by HEW officials for a healthy fee, concluded his criticism of the report by noting that it contained "too much space devoted to defects."

"What end is served?" he asked, implying that defects were useless or inappropriate to mention.

The satisficers were everywhere. An eminent professor, testifying before Congress, was queried by Senator Fred Harris about whether the nation was using all available knowledge to better people's health. Shaking his head with certainty, the professor said that—contrary to popular opinion—there was no problem at all:

> One continues to hear today that there is a great wealth of immediately useful . . . knowledge that the practicing physician . . . is not applying.

"I very much question this notion," the professor concluded.

The very same week that Congress was being assured that every bit of health knowledge that could be used was being utilized, a "progress report" from the Georgia State Health Department crossed my desk. I thumbed through it casually. In the same year in which, according to the professor, every available technique for bettering health was being utilized, the report mentioned the following facts:

> Seven out of eight babies had not received a simple, inexpensive test to detect a treatable cause of mental retardation.

Only one-third of all schoolchildren had their eyes
tested, and half of those who failed the test received
no further care.

Less than one-fifth of all schoolchildren had hearing
tests, and 40 percent of those who failed got no further
care.

The satisficers were everywhere. They were the officials
who said "Our program has been running well enough for
twenty years—why should we make any changes now?" Or
the official who asked, when the Poor People's Campaign
submitted their demands, for a reply that "the Secretary can
live with"—a reply good enough to pacify the poor without
committing HEW to any major changes.

The satisficers were officials who were preoccupied more
with administrative procedures than they were with problems—men who spent their time writing reports full of organ-
izational gobbledygook such as this example from a federal
task force report titled *Health in Housing and Urban Development:*

All relevant . . . program interests and activities must
be integrated and coordinated, and methods of information exchange improved, so as to provide a
strong basis for a consolidated approach to urban . . .
problems.

This sort of bureaucratic "word salad" was evidently
thought, by the official who wrote it, to be good enough to
convince someone that something was going to be done about
the problems of the cities.

"Large bureaucracies," says Henry Rowen, "have remarkable inertia . . . their imperviousness to changes in the exter-
nal environment is often extraordinary."

Most officials whom I met in Washington were scarcely
aware of the inchworm slowness with which the government
moved to face social problems. They were scarcely aware
of the mountains of memoranda that slowly piled up or of

the endless meetings that invariably ended with little or nothing having been accomplished, except an agreement to have some staff member prepare a document to be discussed at the next meeting.

A government official's concept of time, I learned, has little in common with anyone else's. It had taken HEW's officials more than six months to begin a nutrition survey. It took longer to complete some of the reports promised the Poor People's Campaign, let alone do anything about the problems these reports dealt with. It was not uncommon, I found, for memoranda to lie on a bureaucrat's desk for weeks without an answer. It was not uncommon for some to go unanswered at all or to be answered in a barely adequate way.

"I wrote to your department," Congressman Resnick of New York angrily told HEW officials, puzzled at why it was taking so long to start a national survey of hunger and malnutrition. "I asked for this survey. I never got an answer."

The pages of congressional hearings were littered with requests from congressmen to officials—requests that were never answered. Senator Robert Kennedy asked Surgeon General Stewart to devise a program for bringing health services to local areas with serious health problems, including hunger and malnutrition. The late senator asked for recommendations for needed action. No program or recommendations were prepared. Senator Javits asked Secretary Cohen to look into HEW's many formulas for giving federal funds to states and to consider ways in which those formulas—many unchanged for decades—might be made more sensible. No changes were ever suggested.

Even top officials themselves—the secretary or the surgeon general—had trouble getting prompt answers from their subordinates or sometimes any answer at all.

"Do you know what I have to do," one high HEW official told me, "if I want to find out something simple like how many people are on welfare?"

"First," he said, "I have to send a memorandum to the welfare administrator. Then the administrator will send it to the deputy administrator. Then he sends it to the director of program planning and evaluation. He will send it to the bureau chief, who will send it to the division chief, who will send it to the branch chief. Finally the branch chief will send it to one of his staff people.

"And then," he concluded, "it has to come back to me the same way."

"Wouldn't it be easier to just pick up the phone and call direct," I asked.

"Of course," he replied, smiling, "but that's going out of channels."

Actually, the process of going "through channels" had one principal result: it made it easier for officials to satisfice. If a congressman wrote to HEW asking what was being done for hungry children in his district, by the time he got a reply he could hardly help but be satisfied, regardless of how incomplete or incorrect it seemed. If he were not, it would take him days to even find out who had prepared the reply, let alone get anything done to further clarify the situation. The wearisome process of getting information from government agencies could only encourage someone to be content with any answer at all. It could only encourage a top official to be content with the answers sent him by his subordinates, no matter how inadequate these answers might be.

Moreover, an official who went "out of channels" in asking for any sort of information only encouraged the official receiving the request not to reply at all—if he did not wish to —since no official memorandum had ever been received. Occasionally this sort of deliberate nonresponsiveness reached ridiculous proportions. Mary Switzer, one of HEW's chief administrators, refused to prepare a report on a matter pertaining to the Poor People's Campaign because, she claimed, Secretary Cohen had never requested the report in an official written memorandum!

Unfortunately there was virtually nothing any official could do about this sort of situation. As long as a subordinate carried out his job "well enough" even his immediate superior was virtually helpless to get him to do anything he was not inclined to do.

"You know," one elderly bureaucrat told me, "there's nothing the secretary or anybody else can do about how I do my job. Even if they took me up before the Civil Service Review Board, why it'd be three years before any decision would be made, and I'm due to retire before then." This official had risen, by seniority, to the post of assistant to the head of one of HEW's planning offices. Unfortunately, having been trained as a sanitary engineer, he knew absolutely nothing about planning. And, equally unfortunately, he was right—there was nothing anyone, not even the secretary himself, could do to get rid of him.

The government's civil service encouraged this attitude. And within HEW, I soon discovered, there existed another sort of system—a bureaucracy within the bureaucracy—even more stultifying than the regular civil service.

"Do you realize," one young policy analyst, a good friend, said to me, "that you are a member of one of the most anachronistic institutions in the government?"

"The Public Health Service Commissioned Corps," he went on, "is unique among the uniformed services. It has officers, but no men. You're an officer," he said, "even though you don't wear a uniform. But whom do you command? To whom are you responsible?"

I was surprised by what my friend had said. I hadn't really thought much about my status as an "officer." I didn't even own a uniform. There was virtually nothing to distinguish me, or my fellow officers, from the civil servants with whom we worked side by side every day. Many commissioned officers were researchers, working in laboratories, who had obtained their jobs in much the same fortuitous way I had, and who hardly thought of themselves as members of any "uniformed service."

The more I thought about what my friend had said, the more it seemed true. The commissioned corps was a relic from the days when the Public Health Service was more closely connected with the Merchant Marine. Now the corps' only function was to provide young men like myself, who were lucky enough to learn of its existence, with an alternative to service in the Army or in some other branch of the military. The corps was as outdated as the Prussian officer corps. My officer's commission had been granted simply by asking for it, with no proof required that I was more qualified than anyone else for my position—a position I had stumbled upon purely by chance. Despite my officer's rank, I had no responsibility for supervising anyone. To make matters worse, I was responsible, in effect, to no one but the surgeon general himself, who was not even aware of my existence.

Both the commissioned corps and the civil service had certain attributes in common. Both were fairly easy to get into and quite hard to get people out of. I never heard, for example, of a commissioned corps officer being even criticized, let alone dismissed, for failure to do his job. It was almost impossible—as the civil servant had told me—for anyone to be removed from a job, even one which he admitted he couldn't do. Both systems gave automatic promotions and pay raises. Both encouraged incompetence and the incredible slowness with which an agency such as HEW began to react to serious or worsening social problems. Both encouraged the fine bureaucratic art of satisficing.

The more I thought about it, in fact, the more it seemed that a lot that was wrong with the government could be traced to its system of obtaining and retaining employees. There never, for example, seemed to be enough eager, talented people around to do all the things that needed to be done. I found myself many times wishing that I had an entire staff of energetic people to do all the things I would have liked to have done. So short was the government of such people that even summer interns—college students working during their summer recess—could gain a good deal of responsibility merely for the asking.

I was not certain how people of this caliber could be obtained, but I was certain of one thing: the government needed better ways to attract young men and women to work in social programs than the haphazard way in which I had been recruited. A system of recruitment was needed that would give young Americans an opportunity to contribute to the nation's social progress, not by accident but by a thorough search for people who might wish to serve. A system was needed that would seek out young people actively, not just accept those who happened to be fortunate enough to find out about a job opening.

I mentioned my feelings at lunch one day to a group of young people, my fellow workers at HEW.

"What we really need," one replied, "is a system that encourages a commitment to national service, especially for young people."

"We need," said another, "a system that would allow young people to work in some social problem-area of their choice."

We spoke about what such a national service corps might look like. The more we talked, the more excited we became. It might indeed be possible to design a national service corps that matched young people with their choice of career for, say, a two-year period. Such service would not provide an escape from military service for a privileged few, but instead —for those not chosen by random selection for military duty— would provide an opportunity for national and even international service.

The national service corps could, we imagined, be an experiment in social responsibility. Its policies and priorities would be the responsibility of its members to determine and to defend before Congress. Its members could serve in federal, state, or local agencies, and requests from officials in these agencies would be matched with job requests from incoming corps members. Members would be able to join at any time from after high school up to a certain age, perhaps thirty-five, thus assuring that they could bring a wide range of skills and experience to their jobs. The corps could be tied to efforts now already under way such as the Peace Corps or VISTA.

The more we talked, the more such a system seemed possible. If it were set up, not as an escape from military service but as an alternative to it, we agreed, it might attract many young people anxious to work in social programs of various sorts. These people would be bound to have a profound effect on the dozens of federal programs now dominated by old-line officials and old-line ideas. They would provide a much needed infusion of imagination and talent into these agencies.

The national service corps could, we thought, provide the new sorts of people so badly needed in federal social programs.

It could provide people with the skill and the desire to plan social programs. Each of us had seen what passed for planning in the government. We had all seen the four-million-a-minute variety of planning, and the secret budget committee kind. We'd seen how little was known about the magnitude or location of social problems—and how little use officials made of what they did know. We'd seen millions of dollars doled out by formulas, most of which had little or no relevance to social problems—money that never, as a result, quite seemed to reach the people and places where these problems were worst.

There was not, we agreed, likely to be any real planning unless the government could attract more bright, energetic people to try to do it. The national service corps might be able to provide such people.

The corps might provide expediters for our social programs.

There were now so many social programs that practically no one could comprehend them all. Local officials didn't know about programs that could help them. It had taken the city of Oakland, California, several months to find out how many federal programs were operating in the city. Federal officials, in turn, were hopelessly confused about what went on at "the other end of the pipeline." They had no idea, in many cases, of how many people their programs were serving or what sorts of people these were. The people being served were just as confused. A woman living in poverty might receive her health care from one federal program, her job training from another, her child's day care from still another, her food stamps from another, and on and on. It could take her several days just to visit all the agencies that were supposedly trying to assist her.

People were needed to expedite social programs and interpret them to or for people. Perhaps, we thought, a national service corps might attract talent for these tasks.

The corps might provide people to analyze how well our social programs were working. Each of us had seen programs that had been in operation for years without the slightest evidence that they were accomplishing what they had set out to accomplish. Each of us had seen the reams of data collected by federal programs, most of it worthless. Each of us had seen important information, like the computer printouts I had given Robert Choate, which lay unused in the government's files—information that might contain vital clues to the solution of social problems. People were needed who would try to see how well social programs were working and how they might be set on a more accurate course.

Finally, the corps might furnish a vast array of people to work directly with the recipients of federal programs—to work to deliver the services these programs were often failing to deliver, where they were most needed. Teachers, technicians, counselors, physicians, training specialists—there were enough untried experiments in delivering services to people, experiments in human development, to keep thousands of corps members busy. There were enough "results" of past experiments ready for mass application to keep another several thousand occupied.

There was a place for thousands of official "advocates"— people like Walter Gellhorn's ombudsman who could speed the complaints of Americans to Washington. People who could amplify the small, distant expert's voice so that it can be heard in the padded committee rooms of our government advisers. People who could interpret the needs of others—like the marchers of the Poor People's Campaign—to those who were supposed to serve the poor.

"Where will all these people, these corps members, come from?" someone asked.

"They're already here, waiting to be called upon," someone else replied. "Do you know what a returned Peace Corps volunteer told me? 'In Africa,' he said, 'I built an entire hospital myself. I drew the plans, ordered the materials, and supervised the construction. I could never get that kind of responsibility here in the United States.'"

"There are plenty of people if the challenge is there," another agreed.

"Senator Claiborne Pell says than 80 percent of the American work force is engaged in a meaningless job."

"HEW already has 100,000 employees," one girl said. "I'm sure we could design meaningful jobs for three times that number of people."

We continued our discussion of the many types of activities the new service corps might tackle—activities we thought would be meaningful and challenging ones. We built up an impressive inventory of the benefits the service corps could bring.

Suddenly somebody brought us back to reality.

"It would never work. The idea would be too threatening. Congress would look upon it as just another power play—another attempt to set up a huge bureaucracy at their expense."

"There are already too many vested interests," said someone else. "Agencies that are supposed to be doing these sorts of jobs, that would look bad by comparison with a service corps."

"I can just hear Senator Ellender now," said another, "asking what's wrong with the agencies we have already and why we have to create a new agency when there are lots of good ones already available."

"Yes," someone said, "like the Agriculture Department's extension service—teaching all those people in the Mississippi Delta to make better use of the food they don't have the money to buy."

"Can you imagine the Defense Department going for a new manpower system with the power to draw up its own budget plans and to ask Congress for the money? A system in competition with the Selective Service System?"

"Maybe it could work through the Selective Service System. Maybe it could humanize it."

"And what about local officials. They'd never accept corps members. They'd look upon it as just another federal take-over attempt. Remember the fuss over the 'metropolitan expediters' for the model cities' program?"

On and on the criticism went. Most of it, however, was directed toward what faults one or another members of the "power structure" might find with the idea—not to the idea itself. All of us had been around Washington long enough to know that any new idea, however obvious its merits, was bound to be treated with tremendous suspicion by nearly everyone.

"A national service corps," said someone. "The word 'national' is no good. It would also be international, wouldn't it?"

"Good luck," said another, skeptically. "Congress wouldn't even let HEW send a piddling few doctors abroad to work for the Peace Corps. They killed that because the AMA thought they might come back with some socialistic ideas."

"Look at the sanitary engineers. Congress wouldn't even let them work in OEO's poverty centers right here in this country."

The pessimism went on, but each of us knew, at heart, that the germ of the idea was a valid one. We felt that across the nation there were thousands of young people like ourselves, seeking an opportunity to participate in an experiment in social responsibility. Each year thousands of these young people applied for federal summer internships—many more than could be accepted. We knew, or thought we knew, that such an experiment could be devised. And we were certain that, once in operation, it would provide an impetus to our social programs that they could obtain in no other way.

The luncheon group broke up. Our thoughts turned to more immediate problems. But as we all straggled back to our offices, one other advantage to the national service corps idea occurred to me. Such an experiment, I thought, might possibly be a way to provide at least a partial competitor to that peculiar species of individuals now all too ubiquitous in the government's social programs—the satisficers.

# CHAPTER
## 11

## *The Last Decision*

My decision to leave Washington was a gradual one. It grew upon me bit by bit, layer by layer, like the shell of some sea animal. I was influenced by many experiences that had little or nothing to do with my job at HEW, but which reflected a mood in the Capitol that pervaded every agency and consequently affected the feelings of every government employee no matter what his position or purpose.

One evening an elderly lawyer, an old family friend, invited me to his house for dinner. After the meal he led me downstairs to his book-lined study. There he spoke about some of his memories of Washington. He told me of his early career in the government and his dealings with many agencies whose names were only vaguely familiar, agencies that had been the precursors of those I now knew. He spoke of political leaders and officials long since dead. He spoke of the foreign policy predicament in which our present government found itself.

"I remember," he told me, "our experience in the Philippines." The United States, he said, following on the heels of a colonial regime, had waged wars on the Filipino guerrillas. The war was a bitter and brutal one and took our troops into the rough mountains and highlands, with little success. William Howard Taft, the President, came gradually to realize that the guerrillas could not be beaten in this fashion.

"Do you know what Taft decided to do?" this man, who had seen as much Washington history as perhaps anyone in the Capitol, asked me. President Taft, he said, decided to begin a massive construction program in the cities of the Philippines. He withdrew his troops from the mountains. He put them to work on the building program.

"After a while," said my host, "there was no one for the guerrillas to fight. Eventually many of them came to the cities to seek employment in the construction program. And the war just disappeared." The same strategy, he said, could possibly be successful in Vietnam today, but it would take time, first for United States leaders to realize that they could not win the war, and then to put the new strategy into effect.

He asked me about my future plans. I told him that I was undecided as to whether or not to remain in Washington. I asked him for his advice.

Washington, at least for a time, he replied, was not going to be a pleasant place in which to work. More important, life was not going to be very productive for the agencies that "wage peace." There were other problems that would have to be solved first and the energies of Washington's leaders would have to be directed toward solving them. Whatever power could be brought to bear would have to be directed toward the solution of these problems. He paused for a long moment, as though trying to think of a way to summarize a complicated legal argument. Finally he spoke.

"We have lost the ability to influence our government," he said, puffing on his cigar. "And I don't know what can be done about it," he added.

His pessimism was, I felt certain, only transitory. He, like other long-time Washingtonians, would never really lose their influence upon the government, for—in a very real sense —they were part of whatever government was in power. Their skills, built up over years of experience, were needed by the government.

Yet, in another sense, I knew that what he had said was true. The government was destined to be, at least for the time being, one whose entire energies were devoted to the single problem of resolving the war. All other problems were subsidiary. In this single-mindedness, there could be no question of exerting any influence. I had already seen the effects of the war's drain on national resources. I had seen memoranda proposing that a billion dollars be sliced from HEW's new budget, despite the pleas of men like John Gardner that such stupendous cuts were the harbingers of disaster for our domestic programs. I had seen staffs cut back because no money would be available to pay them and new plans scrapped for the same reason.

"It's a good time to leave," said a girl who worked at HEW. "Nothing's going to happen here for a while."

It struck me as strange—the idea that nothing was going to "happen" in a government agency with a budget of some fifteen billion dollars and 100,000 employees. But in a very real sense it was true. Most of HEW's programs, especially those that had been in existence for many years, ran themselves. There was nothing exciting about managing a program that merely doled out money by rote, no matter how important the reason might be for its existence. And there were not likely to be any new programs or, even more important, any major changes in the basic assumptions underlying old ones.

With such a prevailing mood, it was wholly accurate to say that nothing was going to happen at HEW or in any other non-defense agency for a while. Most top officials recognized that this was so. They left in droves: for university posts; for private consulting firms; for nonprofit organizations such as the Urban Coalition; for "think tanks" such as

RAND; for posts in state or local governments; for Washington groups such as the Conference of Mayors; and for a thousand places where, they hoped, something might happen.

I thought for a long time about whether or not to leave Washington. For me, living in the city had been a singular experience. I had grown to love life there. I enjoyed walking down the hill from Georgetown to the concealed circular staircase built into the Francis Scott Key Bridge that led to the river and the canal that ran alongside it. In the evenings I liked going there and standing on the deserted pier of a rowing club, looking out over the river as it turned off into Virginia as though turning its back on the District of Columbia and all the troubles there. I enjoyed ice skating on the canal in winter, between the locks that had not been used for decades.

In Washington I had come in contact with people the likes of whom I'd never met before. The administrator with his cork dartboard who had promised to make me an "expert" overnight. The Episcopalian minister who believed that social progress was a consequence of making the right social policy decisions. Congressional aides wise in the byzantine machinations of getting bills through Congress. Economists who talked about the modified Cobb-Douglas production function as though they expected everyone to know what they meant. Dedicated officials like George Silver who seemed to work night and day just to keep the huge pile of "necessary action" items on their desk at a constant level. Self-taught experts like Robert Choate with an amazing singularity of purpose and energy.

And then, perhaps most important, there had been the experiences—the situations I had seen or in which I'd participated. I felt, in a sense, I'd experienced more perhaps than was salutary for a person my age, that I knew more about the government than would permit me ever again to regard it without a measure of cynicism and even disconsolation.

I had seen more important decisions made—or muddled—than most political scientists would ever see. I'd seen the nub of these decisions, that crucial moment when one man, with the power to influence other men, leans back in his chair and says, "I would blur this issue if at all possible." That crucial moment when one man decides to step back, ever so slightly, from the pursuit of truth and declares that a document contains "too much space devoted to defects."

I had also seen men in their hour of strength. John Gardner, his long legs bent against the desk edge like a man in a rowing machine, summing up a complex issue in a few perfect sentences. Or Wilbur Cohen, when he had just learned of his appointment as HEW's new secretary, his face flushed with the victory of a lifetime, talking eagerly of the things he wanted to accomplish.

There had been moments of incalculable sorrow—watching the cortege of Robert Kennedy pass by Resurrection City, the faces of the poor peering out from between the slats of the snow fence that surrounded the camp. There had been moments of terror—the slowly enlarging cloud billowing behind the Capitol dome on the afternoon of Washington's burning. And there had been humorous moments—the black man who found it hard to believe, looking at Wilbur Cohen, that this "little cat" might be the secretary of HEW.

And there were moments of awe—moments when I felt that an important lesson was about to be imparted and that it was vitally important to acquire as much of it as was humanly possible. Moments, such as my discussion with the lawyer, when I felt I was privileged to catch a glimpse of a part of history that I would never again be able to obtain.

There were, of course, times when I felt that I should remain in Washington—times when I felt the urgency of the many things that remained to be done. In the last days of the Johnson Administration, for example, HEW's Secretary Cohen sent a report to the President that listed the many accomplishments performed by the departing administration, the many new laws that had been passed and the many new programs that had been begun. But the report also told of something else. At its end—almost as an afterthought—the report included a section titled "Goals for 1976." In three short pages some twenty-five specific social goals were listed. These were not the usual vague statements contained in most government reports, statements that Henry Rowen has called "little more than home-and-mother platitudes." These were "hard" goals. The report predicted, for instance, that by 1976 the nation could achieve:

An increase in life expectancy of nearly two years and a decrease of infant mortality by nearly one-half.

Preschool or school participation for virtually all children three to five years old.

Elimination of all American housing units without bath and shower facilities.

Elimination of illiteracy.

An increase from 10.1 to 15 percent in persons who have graduated from college.

An increase of 300 percent in the number of handicapped persons rehabilitated each year.

Many of these goals, I thought while reading the report, looked familiar. I had seen them someplace before. I soon realized why these goals seemed familiar—most of them were borrowed from studies, such as the one dealing with child health that I had helped prepare nearly two years earlier. This study, in turn, was only one of many such analyses dealing with social problems in health, education, job training, and a variety of other areas. In health alone, I realized, HEW had carried out about a half-dozen such analyses. Each of them had contained estimates of possible improvements in the nation's health status. These studies had predicted, for example, that deaths from cancer could be decreased by nearly 100,000 each year; that deaths due to automobile accidents could be cut by probably 10 percent and that deaths due to heart attacks could be diminished by 20 to 30 percent.

These startling predictions were gleaned from the results of successful government-sponsored projects already under way for several years—results that no officials had ever collected in one place before.

In education, for example, the government's billion-dollar program for "disadvantaged" children had been analyzed to see what the results had been. The results showed that disadvantaged children could learn as well as anyone else, given a reasonable amount of teaching effort. Even the most deprived children, the program's results suggested, could learn a year's worth of schooling for every year spent in school—if an adequate effort were made to teach them. The government's analysis had, of course, only confirmed what other, less massive "demonstrations" had already showed. Jonathan Kozol had taken the worst pupils in Boston's Pierce school and in less than a year had transformed them into the best readers in the Boston school system. Herbert Kohl had taken a slow-learning class in Harlem—all of them one to three years behind in reading ability—and had transformed them into a class of eager and expressive young men and women.

Anyone who had worked in the government for a short time could cite numerous other success stories, many supported by federal funds:

An "experiment" in New York City showed that grade school children who received only four hours of tutoring a week gained half a grade in their ability to read.

A "pilot study" in Denver showed that, after a school lunch program was started, school dropouts went down by 37 percent.

A project in Pennsylvania showed that women could be taught, with no special prior training, to do skilled nursing duties in about one-eighth the time usually required.

The U.S. Gypsum Company, in a "demonstration," rehabilitated an entire New York City tenement in only forty-eight hours.

The Head Start program was able to raise the IQs of its "disadvantaged" preschool children by ten points in one summer, and another Government-supported program was able to raise the IQs of infants from "underprivileged" families to better than normal levels after thirty-six months of tutoring.

A West Virginia project increased the incomes of unemployed workers by 40 percent by simply giving them help in relocating to where they could find new jobs.

The Job Corps was able in less than a year to improve the reading ability of its young trainees by one and a half grades, and their arithmetic level by two grades.

HEW's report to President Johnson had taken its goals from dozens of experiences such as these. Someone, probably not an expert but more likely merely someone who had been assigned the job of preparing a report, had taken the trouble to gather together some of these successful projects and to try to predict—based on their results—what it might be possible for the nation as a whole to accomplish.

But hardly any of the officials with whom I worked, I thought—reading HEW's final report—seemed to be interested in looking on a continuing basis for such examples of possible accomplishments. No one seemed to be concerned about finding examples of those things that had already been proven possible and trying to foster their mass application across the country. No one even seemed concerned with drawing up a list of such possible achievements—a national social development plan—for use at some future time.

"There are some things," John Gardner said, after he had left HEW, "that are gravely wrong with our society as a problem-solving mechanism. The machinery of the society is not working in a fashion that will permit us to solve any of our problems effectively."

No one at HEW seemed worried about those "gravely wrong" things. Officials had on their desks computer print-outs, like the one I'd given Robert Choate, that pinpointed the precise localities where schoolchildren were learning less this year than last or where more infants were dying. But no one seemed interested in designing ways for the government to react to such worsening situations. The government was, for all intents and purposes, helpless to react to a rising death rate in Lowndes County, Alabama, increasing welfare rolls in Bedford-Stuyvesant, or worsening air pollution levels in Chicago. And no official seemed interested in doing anything about this impotence.

Officials did not seem interested in finding ways for the government's many agencies to work together to solve social problems. No one, for instance, seemed to wonder if HEW might help locate hungry children for the Agriculture Department's food programs. Or whether our highway construction program could aid our accident prevention program. Or whether our housing program could help our mental health efforts. And on and on.

"I would just like to know," Congresswoman Catherine May of Washington asked federal officials, "why people fall between these programs." None of the officials could give her an answer. They knew that our social programs were designed to deal with people—to borrow Herbert Marcuse's phrase—like one-dimensional men. Our programs, they must have realized, dealt with people like food stamp recipients or day care users or job trainees or unwed mothers—treated them, in other words, as everything but whole people. Yet none of our officials seemed interested in trying to come up with ways to make this situation better. None of them seemed interested in trying to design a framework that might prevent people from falling between the benefits provided by our numerous social programs.

I thought, as I read HEW's list of goals for 1976, of all these things that no official seemed interested in thinking about—these broad questions that concerned the way in which our entire government worked. I knew a young man, for instance, who worked in the surgeon general's planning office and who was interested in developing a framework for social programs to try to eliminate some of the reasons why people and their problems slipped between these efforts. Such a framework would have enabled federal officials to look at the people who were supposed to benefit from their programs as more than one-dimensional people. Unfortunately none of the officials were interested.

"I just don't have the time to think about that sort of thing," said one. "I'm too busy trying to write testimony to explain to Congress why we don't know how many malnourished people there are in the country."

Officials were too busy trying to figure out why a problem like malnutrition—and the people it involved—could fall between the cracks to consider ways to prevent other problems from being overlooked in the future.

There were certainly plenty of unanswered questions and unsolved problems in HEW and in the government at large. They were difficult and worthwhile ones. Yet I felt reasonably certain that none of the top officials were interested in finding the answers. They were too busy worrying whether, with a new administration, their jobs would be in jeopardy. They were too busy worrying about scores of other daily matters. The sorts of questions and problems that I and a few others felt were most crucial did not seem to be of concern to these officials.

From time to time I even wondered whether I was acquiring some of the complacency of the bureaucrats with whom I worked. I occasionally caught myself accepting the sluggish pace of the bureaucracy. I caught myself thinking that, if such-and-such a problem could be made only a little better, it would be adequate for the time being. I caught myself trying to placate men like Bob Choate, and offering lots of reasons to justify why nothing more could be done.

I could not help wonder, as I had wondered before,

whether this was what happened to someone who worked too long in the government. Perhaps he became desensitized to the urgency of things. Perhaps he became satisfied with a good-enough job. Perhaps he finally ceased to be aware of the small, distant voices of people whose daily lives are so intimately affected by the decisions he makes or fails to make.

This disturbing fear—the fear of insidiously acquiring those characteristics I associated with the ineffectualness and unresponsiveness of the government—was just another in a jumble of feelings prompting me to leave Washington. Shortly before I finally did so, I visited the home of a congressional aide with whom I'd become friendly. He had lived, with his family, in the city for several years and had an intimate knowledge of its ways. When I told him I was planning to leave, he looked at me with some surprise.

"Why?" he asked.

I told him, as best I could, of my feelings. I told him of the many important tasks in which I'd participated. I told him of the things that I'd seen muddled or left unfinished— of bureaucratic disasters that affected more Americans than any tornado, earthquake, or hurricane. Disasters that meant the curtailment of life, development, and well-being for nearly everyone. I told him of the things that remained to be done—of the problems none of our officials seemed willing to tackle. I spoke of the all-pervasive attitude that was, I felt certain, a major underlying force in all that is done—or not done—in the government: the attitude that all that is ultimately necessary is to "get by," to do a job that is good enough, to satisfice.

My friend looked at me carefully over the top of his wine goblet. He had also seen, from the perspective of Capitol Hill, many of the same phenomena. He had doubtless seen many others that I knew nothing about. He too, I knew, had toyed with the idea of leaving Washington or at least leaving the government.

"It gets into your blood," he finally said. "You may leave for a while, but you'll be back."

After dinner we walked outside into the fresh Maryland night air. The driveway was unpaved, and there were deep ruts from the last rain. In the back of the house a goat, one of the children's pets, made a suspicious sound. Then there was silence.

"I hope I'll have the driveway paved by the time you return," my host said, smiling.

We shook hands. I got into my car and swung it around, carefully trying to avoid the ruts.

"Perhaps you can get a beautification grant," I said.

Then I left him standing there, kicking one of the ruts, in the deepening darkness.